Obesity - Recent Insights and Therapeutic Options

Edited by Samy I. McFarlane

Published in London, United Kingdom

Obesity - Recent Insights and Therapeutic Options
http://dx.doi.org/10.5772/intechopen.104318
Edited by Samy I. McFarlane

Contributors
Sudipta Chakrabarti, Amina Khatun, Surendra Patra, Kuntal Ghosh, Shrabani Pradhan, Mirjam Močnik, Nataša Marčun Varda, Asad Ullah, Muhammad Jamil, Johar Jamil, Daria Lahoda, Hafeez Abiola Afolabi, Zaidi Zakaria, Salzihan Md. Salleh, Ewe Seng Ch'ng, Siti Norasikin Mohd Nafi, Ahmad Aizat Bin Abdul Aziz, Sameer Badri Al-Mhanna, Abubakar Bishir Daku, Ahmad Adebayo Irekeola, Yusuf Wada, Gitanjali Srivastava, Firas Ghomraoui, Maritza Torres Valdez, Valmore José Bermúdez Pirela, Zaira Dzhamutdinovna Ramazanova, Alexander Sergeevich Ametov, Evgeniya Yurievna Pashkova

First published in London, United Kingdom, 2023 by IntechOpen
IntechOpen is the global imprint of INTECHOPEN LIMITED, registered in England and Wales, registration number: 11086078, 5 Princes Gate Court, London, SW7 2QJ, United Kingdom

British Library Cataloguing-in-Publication Data
A catalogue record for this book is available from the British Library

Additional hard and PDF copies can be obtained from orders@intechopen.com

Obesity - Recent Insights and Therapeutic Options
Edited by Samy I. McFarlane
p. cm.
Print ISBN 978-1-80355-909-4
Online ISBN 978-1-80355-910-0
eBook (PDF) ISBN 978-1-80355-911-7

For EU product safety concerns:
IN TECH d.o.o., Prolaz Marije Krucifikse Kozulić 3, 51000 Rijeka, Croatia,
info@intechopen.com or visit our website at intechopen.com.

Meet the editor

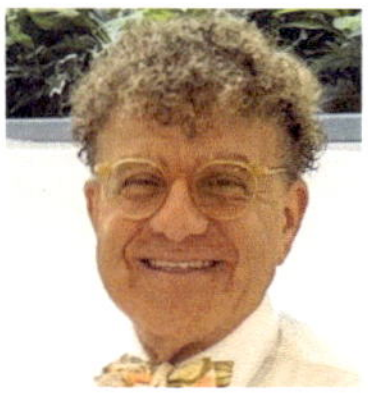

Dr. Samy I. McFarlane is Distinguished Teaching Professor of Medicine/Endocrinology and Associate Dean at Downstate-Health Sciences University, Brooklyn, New York, USA. He has extensive experience in clinical and translational research and served as the principal investigator for the largest center in North America in the landmark Diabetes Reduction Assessment with ramipril and rosiglitazone Medication (DREAM) trial. He has authored more than 400 publications with more than 17,000 citations. Some of his citations are included in major guidelines by the American Heart Association (AHA), such as stroke guidelines (2018 and 2019), the Scientific Statement from the AHA on Lifestyle and Risk Factor Modification for Reduction of Atrial Fibrillation 2020, and the 2021 SHNE/HRS/EHRA/APHRS Expert Collaborative Statement. Most recently, Dr. McFarlane's work was cited by the WHO European Regional Obesity Report 2022. Dr. McFarlane is also the editor of several books on diabetes, hypertension, RAAS, dyslipidemia, cardiovascular disease, and related topics. He is the editor of the study guide, *First Aid for the Medicine Clerkship*, and the *Resident Inpatient Selective Educational (RISE) Manual* (2020 and 2022). Dr. McFarlane is the founding associate editor for *Endocrine Today* and a founding editor in chief, section editor, lead guest editor, and editorial board member for several journals, including *Clinical Practice*, *Current Diabetes Reports*, *Current Hypertension Reports*, *Current Cardiovascular Reports*, *International Journal of Hypertension*, and others. He is a three-term member of the National Institutes of Health-National Institute of Diabetes and Digestive and Kidney Diseases (NIH-NIDDK) and served twice as chair at NIH-NIDDK U01 committees. He also served as chair of the clinical sub-committee of the National Kidney Foundation, Kidney Early Evaluation Program (KEEP). Locally, he held several leadership positions including Director of Internal Medicine Clerkship, Program Director and Chief of Endocrinology, and Medical Director of Clinical Research. He is currently the Internal Medicine Residency Program Director at Downstate-Health Science University, Brooklyn, New York. He also served as Brooklyn District President for the American College of Physicians. Dr. McFarlane is the recipient of numerous awards and honors including recognitions from the United States Army, the US House of Representatives, and the Gold Foundation for Humanism in Medicine, in addition to several teaching and mentoring awards.

Contents

Preface

While the pandemic of obesity continues to affect millions of people around the globe, major developments and insights into the pandemic and pathogenetic mechanisms of obesity-related disorders continue to evolve. Additionally, major developments in the management of obesity continue to progress with rather impressive outcomes.

In this volume, *Obesity – Recent Insights and Therapeutic Options*, we provide the latest developments in the field of obesity in a group of chapters written by experts in the field with direct and intricate knowledge of the disease through research and clinical practice.

Section 1, "Implications of Obesity in Special Populations", includes Chapter 1, "Obesity in Children: Recent Insights and Therapeutic Options" and Chapter 2, "Stigmatization of the Patients Who Live with Overweight or Obesity". The populations discussed in these chapters are particularly vulnerable and suffer from disparities and inequities in health care. However, they are finally gaining attention from health professionals, policy makers, and other stakeholders.

Section 2, "Metabolic and Neurogenic Effects of Obesity: Implications for Chronic Diseases," includes Chapter 3, "Metabolic Changes in Obesity", Chapter 4, "Diet-Induced Overweight Conditions: Effect on Brain Structure, Cognitive Function, and Neurogenesis" and Chapter 5, "Obesity: A Prerequisite for Major Chronic Illnesses".

This section provides current and practical information relevant to our understanding of the pathogenesis of obesity-related disorders.

Finally, Section 3, "Recent Advances and Outcomes of Obesity Management", includes Chapter 6, "Novel Anti-Obesity Pharmacotherapies", Chapter 7, "The Role of Dietary Interventions in the Management of Obesity", and Chapter 8, "Metabolic Outcomes in Obese Patients after Bariatric Embolization of the Left Gastric Vessel". This section discusses recent advances in pharmacology and surgical interventions for obesity as well as presents information regarding the outcomes of these interventions.

This book is timely with useful and practical information that addresses the needs of a variety of readers, including students, busy clinical providers, and researchers alike.

Samy I. McFarlane
Distinguished Teaching Professor of Medicine/Endocrinology and Associate Dean,
Downstate-Health Science University,
United States of America

Section 1

Implications of Obesity in Special Populations

Chapter 1

Obesity in Children: Recent Insights and Therapeutic Options

Mirjam Močnik and Nataša Marčun Varda

Abstract

Obesity in children, including adolescents, is nowadays, in the light of the COVID-19 pandemic, an even more pressing problem than before it, leading to increased prevalence of obesity and its comorbidities at young age. A simple and correct approach to diagnosis is essential, and some new insights in epidemiology, pathophysiology, and diagnosis are currently under investigation. Obesity in preschool children and metabolically healthy obesity are new entities that are recently being defined and written about. Additionally, several new factors that might influence obesity development are being researched, such as pollutants, sleep duration, and gut microbiota. In this chapter, we briefly present them as possible therapeutic targets in the future along with current therapeutic options in the pediatric population, namely lifestyle change, pharmaceutical options, and surgery. A child is always significantly affected by his/her family lifestyle, home, and social environment, which has to be considered in childhood obesity management.

Keywords: obesity, children, adolescents, treatment, recent discoveries

1. Introduction

Obesity, defined by the World Health Organization, as an excess in fat mass great enough to increase the risk of morbidity, altered physical, psychological or social well-being, and/or mortality [1], has reached pandemic proportions in recent decades [2]. Simultaneously, several "adult diseases," such as type 2 diabetes mellitus, hypertension, and nonalcoholic fatty liver disease, are emerging also in the pediatric population, therefore increasing their cardiovascular risk at a young age. Rarely, children can have an underlying endocrine or monogenic cause of their weight gain. Therefore, obesity in childhood is mostly the result of energy intake and expenditure imbalance [2].

In this chapter, we will review some new insights into childhood obesity with possible therapeutic options.

2. Epidemiology

The increasing prevalence of childhood obesity with advancing age is a well-known fact in recent decades and varies by racial, ethnic, and socioeconomic factors [2].

Children of obese parents have an increased risk for obesity development, not only because of hereditary but also due to environmental factors [3]. Additionally, childhood, and especially adolescent obesity, are associated with obesity in adulthood [4, 5], creating a vicious cycle.

After a dramatic increase in obesity prevalence approximately 40 years ago, some studies after the year 2000 showed a steady state; however, these studies were not replicated and a true trend of stabilizing obesity incidence was not proven [2]. Some isolated studies still brought some hope in decreasing obesity in children, but then the COVID-19 pandemic happened and had a significant impact on childhood obesity.

2.1 COVID-19 and obesity in children

The pandemic of childhood obesity has collided with the pandemic of COVID-19 in the last few years [6]. Many countries from all over the world are reporting an increased prevalence of obesity in childhood [7]. Billions of people were subjected to home confinement leading them to change their lifestyles and eating behaviors, including buying and consuming large quantities of preserved and processed food. Simultaneously, sedentary behavior and increased screen time led to decreased physical activity. Isolation, restricted activity, and unhealthy food choices, associated also with financial reasons, are the most commonly identified culprits for increased obesity, along with other psychosocial, behavioral, and environmental factors [6, 7]. Additionally, preexisting disparities in obesity in terms of race, ethnicity, and socioeconomic status increased [8].

3. Etiology and pathophysiology

Obesity in children is usually the consequence of an imbalance between nutrient consumption and energy expenditure, rarely, other causes can be identified. Still, genetic etiology or at least predisposition might play an important role in the pathogenesis of obesity. Genetic predisposition to obesity has been widely accepted; however, there are only few articles associating specific gene pathways to obesity in children, namely Toll-like receptor 4 signaling pathway [9], leptin-melanocortin signaling pathway [10], c-Jun N-terminal kinase signaling pathway [11], and adenosine monophosphate-activated protein kinase signaling pathway [12]. Several genes, however, they were associated with overexpression in visceral fat and subcutaneous adipose tissues, including the phospholipid transfer gene, ras, adipsin, and calcyclin [13, 14] with gene variants associated with severe obesity in both childhood and adulthood [15, 16].

In addition, differentially expressed genes in children with obesity were identified recently in pathways associated with the immune system. Also, matrix metalloproteinase 9 and acetyl-CoA carboxylase ß were identified as hub genes in the protein-protein interaction network and might be marker genes for childhood obesity [17].

Another important association, found recently, is between obesity and sleep deprivation, highlighted by growing evidence, described below. In these studies, autonomic dysfunction is presented as a new possible pathophysiological pathway to obesity development, which was supported by sympathovagal imbalance, particularly during the night in obese children compared to healthy controls [18]; however, the evidence is not conclusive.

DOI: http://dx.doi.org/10.5772/intechopen.108987

4. Diagnosis and risk factors

Evaluation of children with obesity is aimed at determining the diagnosis and the cause of weight gain and assessing for comorbidities resulting from excess weight.

4.1 Establishing the diagnosis

Clinical diagnosis is based on anthropometric measurements, usually widely used as body mass index (BMI). BMI cut-off points in adults (25 and 30 kg/m^2 for overweight and obesity, respectively) are used due to the observed increased health risks at these levels and are adjusted in the pediatric population according to age, sex, and height. BMI has some disadvantages; mainly it does not predict body fat percentage and it does not distinguish between lean and fat mass. Additional measurement of waist/hip circumference is a tool to identify central obesity, associated more strongly with complications, such as insulin resistance, dyslipidemia, and nonalcoholic fatty liver disease [19].

Measuring waist/hip circumference can also be challenging and time-consuming in terms of behavioral, cultural, and environmental issues. Additionally, waist circumference may be affected after eating by abdominal distension. Given these limitations, new strategies to find a better anthropometric obesity measure are evolving. One of them is neck circumference measurement, which has been associated with central obesity and abnormal metabolic status. It can be reliably used to screen overweight and obesity in children with identification of those with high BMI [20, 21].

Interestingly, dermatoglyphic differences have also been observed in children and adolescents with obesity. In participants with normal weight, a higher frequency of ulnar loops on the index and middle finger were noted along with presence of radial loops on the middle finger. In children with obesity, a greater frequency of whorls on the index and middle fingers were observed in males along with arches in the middle finger [22].

Body fat mass can further be estimated by several other methods, namely dual-energy X-ray absorptiometry, bioelectrical impedance assay, computed tomography and magnetic resonance imaging of abdomen, measurement of skinfold thickness at multiple sites, air displacement plethysmography, and stable isotope dilution techniques [19].

4.2 Metabolically healthy obesity in children

Metabolically healthy obesity in children is a new entity mainly regarded as obesity without cardiometabolic risk factors; however, definitions are variable. An international panel of 46 experts agreed that criteria for metabolically healthy obesity in children include high-density lipoprotein-cholesterol >1.03 mmol/l (or > 40 mg/dl), triglycerides ≤1.7 mmol/l (or ≤ 150 mg/dl), systolic and diastolic blood pressure ≤ 90th percentile, and a measure of glycemia [23]. Due to the heterogeneous definition, the prevalence of metabolically healthy obesity varies from 3 to 80% [23]. Specific genetic predispositions and environmental factors or absence (family history, specific gene variants, and decreased physical activity) of them contribute significantly to metabolic health [24]; however, they were not widely researched and accepted yet. It is still unknown if these children have lower cardiovascular risk and can be managed less aggressively.

4.3 Challenges of obesity in children under six years of age

With increasing obesity, preschool years present a point of opportunity for children to be active, develop healthy habits, and maintain a healthy lifestyle, however, the prevalence of obesity in this age group is inconsistent in European countries and varies up to one-third of 5-year-old children. Measuring overweight and obesity in this group may be challenging [25]. The prevalence was lower among children born to parents with high education, and higher among children born to foreign parents and overweight mothers [26].

In younger children with obesity, there is also an increased risk for monogenic or underlying endocrine disease and should be excluded, especially when severe obesity is present. However, in this age group, establishing the diagnosis should be done with caution when obesity is not as severe. It was shown that young children with a high BMI percentile have lower fat mass than older children with the same BMI percentile and therefore obesity in this age group can be over diagnosed [27].

In order to plan appropriate management of obesity in younger children, we need a better understanding of potential modifiable factors. Specific risk factors for obesity in children under six years of age include maternal diabetes, maternal smoking, gestational weight gain, and rapid infant growth [28]. In preschool children, parents can have a significant influence on modifiable risk factors associated with severe obesity already in this age group and also in further growth. These risk factors include inappropriate nutrition (sugar-sweetened beverages and fast food and skipping breakfast), inactivity (low frequency of outdoor play and excessive screen time), behaviors (lower satiety responsiveness, sleeping with a bottle, lack of bedtime rules, and short sleep duration) and socio-environmental risk factors (informal childcare setting, maternal smoking, and maternal obesity) [27, 29].

4.4 Risk factors for obesity development

The development of obesity is very complex and includes many risk factors. Although we mostly define the etiology as an imbalance between calorie intake and consumption, the reality is not as simple. Genetic, biological, and socio-environmental factors, including family, school, community, and national policies, can play a crucial role. The complexity of risk factors among the pediatric population leads to difficulty in treatment and many interventional trials have been proven ineffective [30]. Therefore, early identification of possibly modifiable factors at an individual, local, and global level should be done to allow appropriate management and policies for obesity prevention and treatment.

Traditional risk factors in school children and adolescents include genetic predisposition, diet (fast food and sugar-sweetened food), eating patterns, lack of physical activity and increased sedentary time (viewing television, playing video games, and using computer), unresolved stress, environmental settings (home, school, and community), sociocultural factors [30].

Some new risk factors for obesity development are under investigation and could present a possible modifiable target in obesity management. Additionally, some new insights into already-known risk factors are presented.

4.4.1 Screen time

The relationship between screen time and increased risk of obesity is well documented. Screen media exposure leads to obesity in children and adolescents through increased eating while viewing, increased sedentary time and reduced sleep duration. Randomized controlled trials of reducing screen time in community settings have reduced weight gain in children, demonstrating a cause-and-effect relationship. However, some evidence also suggests a promise for using interactive media to improve eating and physical activity behaviors to prevent or reduce obesity [31].

Studies, reporting associations between obesity and playing video games are almost half positive, and the rest reported no association. There was preliminary evidence on the effectiveness of exergame (physically active) play for weight reduction and to attenuate weight gain; however, there was little indication that interventions effectively reduced video game play or general screen time [32].

4.4.2 Obesity and sleep duration

The present studies indicate that short sleep duration increases the risk of childhood obesity, making appropriate sleep duration another priority in a child's life [33, 34]. Few studies examined other dimensions of sleep, namely quality, efficiency, and bed/wake time in association with weight status. Even when present, there were variations in defining and measuring these dimensions, making their comparison and potential discrepancies difficult to assess [35].

There are several mechanisms proposed to link sleep loss and the risk of weight gain, based on hormonal and neuroendocrine changes associated with sleep restriction. One of the potential may lie within the hypothalamus or within hypothalamic communication with the peripheral system, and through hormonal systems via leptin and ghrelin (with peripheral metabolic indicators, such as glucose and cholecystokinin). Two distinct neuropeptides, orexin A in B, are synthesized mainly by the neurons in some parts of the hypothalamus and are believed to play a key role in the interaction between sleep and feeding. Orexins induce and support arousal and promote feeding, and are involved in the regulation of many functions, such as sleep-wakefulness, locomotor activity, feeding, thermoregulation, and neuroendocrine and cardiovascular control. Orexin neurons may be disinhibited by low levels of leptin and glucose and excited by ghrelin. Orexin activity is associated with an increased sympathetic tone, which in sleep deprivation may further inhibit leptin release and stimulate ghrelin release, consistent with the effects of short sleep on the peripheral levels of both hormones already observed in adult population [36]. Increased catecholamine levels in sleep deprivation also inhibit insulin secretion and promote glycogen breakdown, increasing the risk of hyperglycemia and insulin resistance seen in obesity [36]. Additionally, it has been suggested that C-reactive protein (CRP) is a leptin-binding protein, and increased CRP levels, seen in obesity, could present a possible mechanism for leptin resistance [36]. There may also be a role for the reward system in modulating food intake and energy storage following a state of sleep loss. Voluntary sleep restriction has been shown to increase snacking, the number of meals eaten per day, and the preference for energy-dense foods [37]. Decreased sleep may also have an adverse effect on energy expenditure. It is also possible that behavioral changes and poor parent-child dynamics may influence sleep deprivation in children, contributing further to weight gain, present already due to other socioeconomic factors [36].

4.4.3 Obesity and gut microbiota

Antibiotics are one of the most commonly prescribed drugs in childhood and their use can cause unwanted problems. Among these, antibiotic-induced gut microbiota dysbiosis has been associated with obesity. This problem is even more relevant to children that are frequently treated with antibiotics. The microbiota composition and its disturbance in neonatal and in early childhood have a profound impact further in life. It can contribute to a decrease in the number and composition of microbiomes affecting glucose and lipid metabolism and immune system development [38]. Evidence suggests that short-chain fatty acids made by the gut microbiota directly or indirectly modulate physiological and pathological processes in relation to obesity. At first glance, excessive short-chain fatty acids represent an additional energy source and could cause an imbalance in energy regulation. Simultaneously, however, short-chain fatty acids participate in glucose-stimulated insulin secretion and release of peptide hormones, which control appetite [39]. However, the causal effect has not been defined and no definitive therapeutic approach has been elucidated. Probiotics and prebiotics could play a role in treating microbial dysbiosis. The addition of specific bacterial strains has been associated with normal weight gain [38]. Dietary modulation has been proven effective also in children with genetic obesity [40].

The exact microbiota status in obesity has not been elucidated yet; however, some studies have tackled this challenge. One study showed associations between *Firmicutes spp*. to obesity and *Bifidobacterium spp*. with a healthy weight in children [41]. Additionally, the addition of *Lactobacillus casei* strain was associated with weight loss while also improving lipid metabolism in obese children via significant increase in the fecal *Bifidobacterium* numbers [42].

4.4.4 Obesity and pollutants

Due to the increase in pollutants in our environment, their concentration has been associated with childhood obesity several times. Recent meta-analyses showed that air pollution is correlated with a substantially increased risk of childhood obesity [43, 44]. The biological and physiological mechanisms regarding the cause-and-effect between air pollution and obesity are still unclear [43]. Animal studies showed that ambient air pollution exaggerated adipose inflammation and insulin resistance [45]. This may further affect the basal metabolic rate and appetite control of exposed individuals [43]. Another animal experiment indicated that exposure to air pollution results in Toll-like receptor 2/4-dependent inflammatory activation in lipid oxidation could lead to metabolic dysfunction and weight gain [46]. Air pollution might also prevent people from going out, causing excess sedentary time, especially in some heavily polluted parts of the world [43].

Along with pollution, other chemicals may affect obesity development. They are called obesogens and are defined as exogenous chemicals belonging to the group of endocrine-disrupting chemicals and are believed to interfere with obesity development. The major mechanism through which obesogens can contribute to obesity is believed to be the activation of nuclear receptors involved in adipogenesis, lipid metabolism, inflammation, and maintenance of metabolic homeostasis. Several chemicals are under investigation as potential causal factors in obesity development; however, these associations remain controversial and it is difficult to find evidence for direct causality between environmental exposure and disease [47]. These chemicals include bisphenol A [47], phthalates [48], perfluoroalkyl substances [49], polycyclic aromatic hydrocarbons [50, 51], etc.

5. Obesity prevention

Disease prevention is even more important in obesity since there are numerous complications, presented in **Table 1**, associated with obesity and even more pronounced when obesity is present early in life [30].

Obesity prevention is therefore a major challenge that has yet to be tackled appropriately. So far, the success of our intervention showed that our understanding of effective prevention is still not achieved [52].

Preventive activity is divided into primordial, primary, secondary, and tertiary. It is primarily achieved by implementing measures to ensure a normal weight and health, and prevent the development of obesity. Public health and national policy strategies play an important role in primordial prevention. The approaches are cost-effective and reduce the overall burden of obesity. With primary prevention, we want to eliminate or reduce exposure to all factors that cause obesity. Effective secondary prevention of obesity is based on early detection and population screening. Tertiary prevention strategies are focused on reducing or delaying the long-term complications that can be caused by obesity (**Table 1**) [53, 54].

Our understanding of childhood obesity, energy balance-related behaviors, determinants of behavior, and effective components of prevention programs is still deficient [52]. Mostly, interventions consist of diet combined with physical activity at individual or community level. Combined interventions had moderate success in children younger than 5 years; however, weaker evidence is present with only dietary or only physical activity interventions [55]. In contrast, in older children, interventions focused only on physical activity can reduce the risk of obesity, but there is no evidence that interventions focused only on diet are effective. Importantly, combined diet and exercise might prove more effective; however, behavioral prevention programs were associated with small improvements in weight outcomes [55, 56].

Cardiovascular	dyslipidaemia, hypertension, left ventricular hypertrophy, coagulopathy, chronic inflammation, endothelial dysfunction
Pulmonary	obstructive sleep apnea, asthma, exercise intolerance
Gastrointestinal	gastroesophageal reflux, non-alcoholic fatty liver disease, steatohepatitis, gallstones, constipation
Endocrine	insulin resistance, type 2 diabetes, precocious puberty, polycystic ovary syndrome (girls), hypogonadism (boys)
Renal	glomerulosclerosis
Neurological	idiopathic intracranial hypertension (pseudotumour cerebri)
Dermatologic	acanthosis nigricans, intertrigo, hidradenitis suppurativa, furunculosis, stretch marks
Musculoskeletal	slipped capital femoral epiphysis, Blount's disease, forearm fracture, back pain, flat feet
Psychosocial	poor self-esteem, anxiety, depression, eating disorders, social isolation, lower educational attainment
Long-term risks	carotid artery atherosclerosis, colorectal carcinoma, ischemic heart disease, stroke, short life span, premature death

Table 1.
Complications of childhood and adolescent obesity [30].

6. Therapeutic options

Obesity management in childhood is based on lifestyle interventions with an emphasis on dietary and physical activity modifications, possibly involving the whole family. However, only a modest effect of lifestyle interventions is seen in severe obesity [57], requiring a consideration about which therapeutic approach to use according to the severity of obesity and the presence of obesity-related comorbidities. Pharmaceutical and surgical options are limited, as presented below.

6.1 Lifestyle interventions

Lifestyle interventions include behavioral measures to alter dietary habits and increase physical activity and are the preferred methods to treat overweight and obesity in children and adolescents. A variety of multicomponent lifestyle interventions may improve BMI in children and adolescents with varying degrees of overweight and obesity [57]. Commonly, they have produced losses from 5 to 20% of excess weight over 3 to 6 months in children [58]. Over 6 to 12 months, the change has ranged from 25% loss to 10% increase in excess weight [58]. In children up to the age of 6 years, a reduction in BMI Z-scores up to 2-year follow-up showed beneficial effects of diet, physical activity, and behavioral interventions. In older children, the beneficial effect of the same measures was found in at least of 6 months of interventions duration [59]. The durability of weight loss is often limited by physiologic systems that are evolutionarily designed to promote weight gain, making lifestyle interventions even more difficult. Continued treatment preventing relapse with face-to-face interventions with a multidisciplinary approach is recommended [60].

Physical activity of at least 60 minutes a day at a moderate-vigorous level is usually recommended [61]. Dietary approaches to weight loss focus on caloric restriction with limited guidelines recommending a very low-carbohydrate/ketogenic diet. Dietary approaches beyond simply caloric restriction with individual assessment and care are recommended for optimal patient outcomes [62]. Additionally, eating behavior has an important impact on obesity development. It was shown that skipping breakfast in the family had significantly increased the risk of childhood overweight and obesity [63]. The same applies to high-energy intake at dinner or late-night snacking [64].

Children that were breastfed for at least 12 months had a significantly lower risk of being overweight or obese than those breastfed for less than 17 weeks. The age of introduction of solid food was not associated with the risk of excess weight at 2 or 3 years of age [65]. Interestingly, dairy products consumption later in life has also been associated with decreased risk of obesity [66].

Not only the amount but also the composition of food intake is of crucial importance. Despite the increased intake, children with obesity often exhibit vitamin D deficiency, usually associated with decreased outdoor activities [67, 68], making appropriate dietary management even more demanding.

All lifestyle interventions should be supported by psychosocial support and treatment that are carried out simultaneously to achieve maximal success. Well-established psychological treatments include family-based behavioral treatment and parent-only behavioral treatment for children utilizing behavioral strategies. Appetite awareness training and regulation of cues treatments are considered experimental. Additional research is needed to test a stepped care model for treatment and to establish the ideal dosage (number and length of the sessions), duration, and intensity of treatments for long-term sustainability of healthy weight management [69].

Especially in severe obesity, lifestyle changes alone, although of fundamental importance, are frequently insufficient. Drug therapies for children are limited and surgical approaches associated with potential morbidity have less known long-term consequences. However, for children with severe obesity, a multifaceted behavioral, pharmacological and surgical approach may be implemented [70].

6.2 Pharmaceutical options

The current use of pharmacotherapy for the treatment of obesity in the pediatric population is limited. Several anti-obesity medications have been approved by the Food and Drug Administration for use among adult patients; however, they are used off-label in the pediatric population [71]. Most commonly prescribed drugs include metformin, topiramate, sibutramine, orlistat, and combinations with fluoxetine and exenatide [71, 72]. A systematic review showed that pharmacological interventions using metformin, sibutramin, orlistat, or fluoxetine may have small effects on BMI reduction. However, trials conducted were generally of low quality, with many having a short or no post-intervention follow-up period and high dropout rates. Adverse effects have also been reported but not in a standardized manner [72]. Therefore, the current endocrine society practice guidelines recommend that these drugs should be used only in clinical trials [73] and only orlistat for patients older than 12 years of age, and phentermine in those older than 16 years are currently approved by the Food and Drug Administration [71, 74].

6.3 Surgical options

The most commonly known surgical option is bariatric surgery, which has been shown to result in a significant and sustained decrease in BMI and improved comorbidities in adult patients. In the pediatric population, there has been an increase in bariatric surgery use, although it is still infrequently performed. Several types of bariatric surgery are being used, most commonly laparoscopic sleeve gastrectomy and Roux-en-Y gastric bypass. The first one carries a lower risk of micronutrient deficiencies (the procedure does not result in malabsorption) and is less complex to do. The Roux-en-Y gastric bypass results in restriction of caloric intake (reduced capacity and neuroendocrine mechanisms) and malabsorption of food along with vitamins and minerals [2]. Adjustable gastric banding is also done in adolescents. Appropriate patient selection is of utmost importance, and the following criteria have been developed [modified according to references 2 and 75]:

1. Body mass index >35 kg/m^2 and a severe comorbidity,

2. Physical maturity (completing 95% of predicted adult stature based on bone age or reaching Tanner stage IV),

3. History of lifestyle changes to lose weight,

4. Ability and motivation of the patient and family to adhere to pre- and postoperative treatments,

5. Understanding of the risks and benefits of surgery,

6. Family support [2, 75].

Contraindications are rare but include a medically correctable cause of obesity, a medical, psychiatric, psychosocial, or cognitive condition that prevents adherence to postoperative dietary and medication regimens, current or planned pregnancy within 12 to 18 months of the procedure, an inability on the part of the patient or parent to comprehend the risks and benefits of the surgical procedure and an ongoing substance abuse problem [75]. Short-term complications include wound infections, leakage at anastomotic sites, pulmonary embolism, small bowel obstruction, gastrojejunal strictures, and gastrogastric fistula. Long-term complications include nutritional deficiencies of iron, vitamin B12, thiamine, and vitamin D. Lifelong vitamin and mineral supplementation is recommended to prevent the development of nutritional deficiencies as a result of decreased intake or malabsorption [2].

According to research, adolescents reached similar weight loss benefits as adults five years after gastric bypass surgery. Improvements in diabetes and hypertension were even greater than in adults [76].

Another possibility is endoscopic procedures, such as an intragastric balloon, for a limited period of time as an adjunct, which showed good efficacy in weight loss and comorbidities improvement with a good safety profile [76].

7. Psychosocial and parental influence

When managing behavioral changes in children, psychosocial and parental factors have to be considered as two elements necessary for effective management.

Childhood is regarded as the most important period of life affecting adulthood. Health problems or illnesses during this period would be brought to maturity or become a risk factor for the onset of diseases in adulthood [77]. The family and environment provide a great impact on social, cognitive, behavioral, and health aspects, including overweight and obesity. Interventions in this field should begin in childhood. Parents play a critical role in shaping child's healthy lifestyle from an early age. They should pay attention to children's weight, eating behavior, and food intake. They are also role models for their children. With their involvement, the long-term effects of lifestyle interventions are enhanced. The most effective way of preventing and controlling overweight and obesity is through family empowerment, including parental knowledge about nutrition, its influence on food choice, eating patterns, sedentary habits, and physical activity. The beliefs and parent's lifestyle and health promotion are also of vital importance due to learning by imitation [77]. Interestingly, parent-only interventions had a similar effect compared with parent-child interventions in children 5 to 11 years [78].

Several socioeconomic factors also influence obesity development in multifaceted ways from an early age on and should be accounted for in childhood obesity management [79, 80].

8. Conclusions

Obesity in children is a significant medical problem, leading to several comorbidities. Several new insights are being researched in diagnosis, management, and treatment options. Additionally, several new factors that might influence obesity development are being identified and researched, such as pollutants, sleep duration, and gut microbiota. In this chapter, we briefly presented them as a possible therapeutic target in the future along with current therapeutic options in the pediatric population, namely lifestyle change, pharmaceutical, and surgical options. A child is always significantly affected by his/her family lifestyle, home, and social environment, which has to be considered in child obesity management.

Conflict of interest

The authors declare no conflict of interest.

Author details

Mirjam Močnik[1]* and Nataša Marčun Varda[2]

1 Department of Pediatrics, University Medical Center Maribor, Maribor, Slovenia

2 Department of Pediatrics, University Medical Center Maribor and Medical Faculty, University of Maribor, Maribor, Slovenia

*Address all correspondence to: mirjammocnik91@gmail.com

References

[1] WHO Technical Consultation. Obesity: Preventing and managing the global epidemic. In: Report of a WHO Consultation 2000. Report No.: 0512-3054 (Print) 0512-3054, 2000. Geneva: WHO; 2000

[2] Kumar S, Kelly AS. Review of childhood obesity: From epidemiology, etiology, and comorbidities to clinical assessment and treatment. Mayo Clinic Proceedings. 2017;**92**:251-265. DOI: 10.1016/j.mayocp.2016.09.017

[3] Whitaker RC, Wright JA, Pepe MS, Seidel KD, Dietz WH. Predicting obesity in young adulthood from childhood and parental obesity. New England Journal of Medicine. 1997;**337**:869-873. DOI: 10.1056/NEJM199709253371301

[4] Parsons TJ, Power C, Logan S, Summerbell CD. Childhood predictors of adult obesity: A systematic review. International Journal of Obesity and Related Metabolic Disorders. 1999;**23**: S1-S107

[5] Ogden CL, Flegal KM, Carroll MD, Johnson CL. Prevalence and trends in overweight among US children and adolescents, 1999-2000. Journal of the American Medical Association. 2002;**288**:1728-1732. DOI: 10.1001/jama.288.14.1728

[6] Tsenoli M, Smith JEM, Khan MAB. A community perspective of COVID-19 and obesity in children: Causes and consequences. Obesity Medicine. 2021;**22**:100327. DOI: doi.org/10.1016/j.obmed.2021.100327

[7] Stavridou A, Kapsali E, Panagouli E, Thirios A, Polychronis K, Bacopoulou F, et al. Obesity in children and adolescents during COVID-19 pandemic. Children (Basel). 2021;**8**:135. DOI: 10.3390/children80220135

[8] Jenssen BP, Kelly MK, Powell M, Bouchelle Z, Mayne SL, Fiks AG. COVID-19 and changes in child obesity. Pediatrics. 2021;**147**:e2021050123. DOI: 10.1542/peds.2021-050123

[9] KIM KA, Gu W, Lee IA, Joh EH, Kim DH. High fat diet-induced gut microbiota exacerbates inflammation and obesity in mice via the TLR4 signalling pathway. PLoS One 2012;7:e47713. DOI: 10.1371/journal.pone.0047713

[10] Farooqi IS, O'Rahilly S. Mutations in ligands and receptors of the leptin-melanocortin pathway that lead to obesity. Nature Clinical Practice. Endocrinology & Metabolism. 2008;**4**:569-577. DOI: 10.1038/ncpendmet0966

[11] Vernia S, Cavanagh-Kyros J, Barrett T, Jung DY, Kim JK, Davis RJ. Diet-induced obesity mediated by the JNK/DIO2 signal transduction pathway. Genes & Development. 2013;**27**:2345-2355. DOI: 10.1101/gad.223800.113

[12] Hwang JT, Kim SH, Lee MS, Kim SH, Yang HJ, Kim MJ, et al. Anti-obesity effects of ginsenoside Rh2 are associated with the activation of AMPK signalling pathway in 3T3-L1 adipocyte. Biochemical and Biophysical Research Communications. 2007;**364**:1002-1008. DOI: 10.1016/j.bbrc.2007.10.125

[13] Vohl MC, Sladek R, Robitaille J, Gurd S, Marceau P, Richard D, et al. A survey of genes differentially expressed in subcutaneous and visceral adipose tissue in men. Obesity Research. 2004;**12**:1217-1222. DOI: 10.1038/oby.2004.153

[14] Linder K, Arner P, Flores-Morales A, Tollet-Egnell P, Norstedt G. Differentially expressed genes in visceral or subcutaneous adipose tissue of obese men and women. Journal of Lipid Research. 2004;**45**:148-154. DOI: 10.1194/jlr.M300256-JLR200

[15] Frayling TM, Timpson NJ, Weedon MN, Zeggini E, Freathy RM, Lindgren CM, et al. A common variant in the FTO gene is associated with body mass index and predisposes to childhood and adult obesity. Science. 2007;**316**:889-894. DOI: 10.1126/science.1141634

[16] Dina C, Meyre D, Gallina S, Durand E, Körner A, Jacobson P, et al. Variation in FTO contributes to childhood obesity and severe adult obesity. Nature Genetics. 2007;**39**: 724-726. DOI: 10.1038/ng2048

[17] Li L, Wang G, Li N, Yu H, Si J, Wang J. Identification of key genes and pathways associated with obesity in children. Experimental and Therapeutic Medicine. 2017;**14**:1065-1073. DOI: 10.3892/etm.2017.4597

[18] Jarrin DC, JJ MG, Poirier P, Quality Cohort Collaborative Group. Autonomic dysfunction: A possible pathophysiological pathway underlying the association between sleep and obesity in children at-risk for obesity. Journal of Youth and Adolescence. 2015;**44**:285-297. DOI: 10.1007/s10964-014-0235-3

[19] Aggarwal B, Jain V. Obesity in children: Definition, etiology and approach. Indian Journal of Pediatrics. 2018;**85**:463-471. DOI: 10.1007/s12098-017-2531-x

[20] Taheri M, Kajbaf TZ, Taheri MR, Aminzadeh M. Neck circumference as a useful marker for screening overweight and obesity in children and adolescents. Oman Medical Journal. 2016;**31**:170-175. DOI: 10.5001/omj.2016.34

[21] Payab M, Qorbani M, Shahbal N, Motlagh ME, Hasani-Ranjbar S, Kelishadi R. Association of anthropometric indices with metabolic phenotypes of obesity in children and adolescents: The CASPIAN-V study. Frontiers in Endocrinology (Lausanne). 2019;**10**:786. DOI: 10.3389/fendo.2019.00786

[22] Alberti A, Ruiz Reyes MA, De Jesus JA, Rossoni C, Grigollo L, Da Silva BB, et al. Identification of obesity in children and teenagers. Minerva Pediatrica. 2021. DOI: 10.23736/S0026-4946.20.05731-X [Online ahead of print]

[23] Damanhoury S, Newton AS, Rashid M, Hartling L, Byrne JLS, Ball GDC. Defining metabolically healthy obesity in children: A scoping review. Obesity Reviews. 2018;**19**:1476-1491. DOI: 10.1111/obr.12721

[24] Li L, Yin J, Cheng H, Wang Y, Gao S, Li M, et al. Identification of genetic and environmental factors predicting metabolically healthy obesity in children: Data from the BCAMS study. The Journal of Clinical Endocrinology and Metabolism. 2016;**101**:1816-1825. DOI: 10.1210/jc.2015-3760

[25] Jones RE, Jewell J, Saksena R, Ramos Salas X, Breda J. Overweight and obesity in children under 5 years: Surveillance opportunities and challenges for the WHO European region. Frontiers in Public Health. 2017;**5**:58. DOI: 10.3389/fpubh.2017.00058

[26] Paduano S, Borsari L, Salvia C, Arletti S, Tripodi A, Pinca J, et al. Risk factors for overweight and obesity in children attending the first year of primary schools in Modena, Italy. Journal of Community Health. 2020;**45**:301-309. DOI: 10.1007/s10900-019-00741-7

[27] Wright CM, Cole TJ, Fewtrell M, Williams JE, Eaton S, Wells JC. Body

composition data show that high BMI centiles overdiagnose obesity in children aged under 6 years. The American Journal of Clinical Nutrition. 2022;**116**:122-131. DOI: 10.1093/ajcn/nqub421

[28] US Preventive Services Task Force, Grossman DC, Bibbins-Domingo K, Curry SJ, Barry MJ, Davidson KW, et al. Screening for obesity in children and adolescents: US preventive services task force recommendation statement. Journal of the American Medical Association. 2017;**317**:2417-2426. DOI: 10.1001/jama.2017.6803

[29] Porter RM, Tindall A, Gaffka BJ, Kirk S, Santos M, Abraham-Pratt I, et al. A review of modifiable risk factors for severe obesity in children ages 5 and under. Childhood Obesity. 2018;**14**:468-476. DOI: 10.1089/chi.2017.0344

[30] Lee EY, Yoon KH. Epidemic obesity in children and adolescents: Risk factors and prevention. Frontiers in Medicine. 2018;**12**:658-666. DOI: 10.1007/s11684-018-0640-1

[31] Robinson TN, Banda JA, Hale L, Lu AS, Fleming-Milici F, Calvert SL, et al. Screen media exposure and obesity in children and adolescents. Pediatrics. 2017;**140**:S97-S101. DOI: 10.1542/peds.2016-1758K

[32] Kracht CL, Joseph ED, Staiano AE. Video games, obesity and children. Current Obesity Reports. 2020;**9**:1-14. DOI: 10.1007/s13679-020-00368-z

[33] Li L, Zhang S, Huang Y, Chen K. Sleep duration and obesity in children: A systematic review and meta-analysis of prospective cohort studies. Journal of Paediatrics and Child Health. 2017;**53**:378-385. DOI: 10.1111/jpc.13434

[34] Fatima Y, Doi SA, Mamun AA. Longitudinal impact of sleep on overweight and obesity in children and adolescents: A systematic review and bias-adjusted meta-analysis. Obesity Reviews. 2015;**16**:137-149. DOI: 10.1111/obr.12245

[35] Morrissey B, Taveras E, Allender S, Strugnell C. Sleep and obesity among children: A systematic review of multiple sleep dimensions. Pediatric Obesity. 2020;**15**:e12619. DOI: 10.1111/ijpo.12619

[36] Hanlon EC, Dumin M, Pannain S. Chapter 13 - sleep and obesity in children and adolescents. In: Bagchi D, editor. Global Perspectives on Childhood Obesity. 2nd ed. Cambridge, Massachusetts: Academic Press; 2019. pp. 147-178. DOI: 10.1016/B978-0-12-812840-4.00013-X

[37] Chaput JP. Is sleep deprivation a contributor to obesity in children? Eating and Weight Disorders. 2016;**21**:5-11. DOI: 10.1007/s40519-015-0233-9

[38] Principi N, Esposito S. Antibiotic administration and the development of obesity in children. International Journal of Antimicrobial Agents. 2016;**47**:171-177. DOI: 10.1016/j.ijantimicag.2015.12.017

[39] Murugesan S, Nirmalkar K, Hoyo-Vadillo C, García-Espitia M, Ramírez-Sánchez D, García-Mena J. Gut microbiome production of short-chain fatty acids and obesity in children. European Journal of Clinical Microbiology & Infectious Diseases. 2018;**37**:621-625. DOI: 10.1007/s10096-017-3143-0

[40] Zhang C, Yin A, Li H, Wang R, Wu G, Shen J, et al. Dietary modulation of gut microbiota contributes to alleviation of both genetic and simple obesity in children. eBioMedicine. 2015;**2**:968-984. DOI: 10.1016/j.ebiom.2015.07.007

[41] Da Silva CC, Monteil MA, Davis EM. Overweight and obesity in children are associated with an abundance of Firmicutes and reduction of Bifidobacterium in their gastrointestinal microbiota. Childhood Obesity. 2020;**16**:204-210. DOI: 10.1089/chi.2019.0280

[42] Nagata S, Chiba Y, Wang C, Yamashiro Y. The effects of the lactobacillus casei strain on obesity in children: A pilot study. Beneficial Microbes. 2017;**8**:535-543. DOI: 10.3920/BM2016.0170

[43] Guo Q, Xue T, Jia C, Wang B, Cao S, Zhao X, et al. Association between exposure to fine particulate matter and obesity in children: A national representative cross-sectional study in China. Environment International. 2020;**143**:105950. DOI: 10.1016/j.envint.2020.105950

[44] Parasin N, Amnuaylojaroen T, Saokaew S. Effect of air pollution on obesity in children: A systematic review and meta-analysis. Children (Basel). 2021;**8**:327. DOI: 10.3390/children8050327

[45] Sun Q, Yue P, Deiuliis JA, Lumeng CN, Kampfrath T, Nikolaj MB, et al. Ambient air pollution exaggerates adipose inflammation and insulin resistance in a mouse model of diet-induced obesity. Circulation. 2009;**119**:538-546. DOI: 10.1161/CIRCULATIONAHA.108.799015

[46] Wei Y, Zhang JJ, Li Z, Gow A, Chung KF, Hu M, et al. Chronic exposure to air pollution particles increases the risk of obesity and metabolic syndrome: Findings from a natural experiment in Beijing. The FASEB Journal. 2016;**30**:2115-2122. DOI: 10.1096/fj.201500142

[47] Kim KY, Lee E, Kim Y. The association between bisphenol a exposure and obesity in children - a systematic review with meta-analysis. International Journal of Environmental Research and Public Health. 2019;**16**:2521. DOI: 10.3390/ijerph16142521

[48] Amin MM, Ebrahimpour K, Parastar S, Shoshtari-Yeganeh B, Hashemi M, Mansourian M, et al. Association of urinary concentrations of phthalate metabolites with cardiometabolic risk factors and obesity in children and adolescents. Chemosphere. 2018;**211**:547-556. DOI: 10.1016/j.chemosphere.2018.07.172

[49] Geiger SD, Yao P, Vaughn MG, Qian Z. PFAS exposure and overweight/obesity among children in a nationally representative sample. Chemosphere. 2021;**268**:128852. DOI: 10.1016/j.chemosphere.202.128852

[50] Bushnik T, Wong SL, Holloway AC, Thomson EM. Association of urinary polycyclic aromatic hydrocarbons and obesity in children aged 3-18: Canadian health measures survey 2009-2015. Journal of Developmental Origins of Health and Disease. 2020;**11**:623-631. DOI: 10.1017/S2040174419000825

[51] Poursafa P, Dadvand P, Amin MM, Hajizadeh Y, Ebrahimpour K, Mansourian M, et al. Association of polycyclic aromatic hydrocarbons with cardiometabolic risk factors and obesity in children. Environment International. 2018;**118**:203-210. DOI: 10.1016/j.envint.2018.05.048

[52] Visscher TL, Kremers SP. How can we better prevent obesity in children? Current Obesity Reports. 2015;**4**:371-378. DOI: 10.1007/s13679-015-0167-6

[53] Patel SS, Daniels SR. Beginning with the end in mind: The case for primordial

and primary cardiovascular prevention in the youth. The Canadian Journal of Cardiology. 2020;**36**:1344-1351. DOI: 10.1016/j.cjca.2020.07.002

[54] Lancarotte I, Nobre MR. Primordial and primary prevention programs for cardiovascular diseases: From risk assessment through risk communication to risk reduction. A review of the literature. Clinics (Sao Paolo). 2016;**71**:667-678. DOI: 10.6061/clinics/2016(11)09

[55] Brown T, Moore TH, Hooper L, Gao Y, Zayegh A, Ijaz S, et al. Interventions for preventing obesity in children. Cochrane Database of Systematic Reviews. 2019;7:CD001871. DOI: 10.1002/12651858.CD001871.pub4

[56] Peirson L, Fitzpatrick-Lewis D, Morrison K, Ciliska D, Kenny M, Usman Ali M, et al. Prevention of overweight and obesity in children and youth: A systematic review and meta-analysis. CMAJ Open. 2015;**3**:E23-E33. DOI: 10.9778/cmajo.20140053

[57] Elvsaas IKO, Giske L, Fure B, Juvet LK. Multicomponent lifestyle interventions for treating overweight and obesity in children and adolescents: A systematic review and meta-analyses. Journal of Obesity. 2017;**2017**:5021902. DOI: 10.1155/2017/5021902

[58] Dietz WH, Robinson TN. Clinical practice. Overweight children and adolescents. The New England Journal of Medicine. 2005;**352**:2100-2109. DOI: 10.1056/NEJMcp043052

[59] Colquitt JL, Loveman E, O'Malley C, Azevedo LB, Mead E, Al-Khudairy L, et al. Diet, physical activity, and behavioural interventions for the treatment of overweight or obesity in preschool children up to the age of 6 years. Cochrane Database of Systematic Reviews. 2016;**3**:CD012105. DOI: 10.1002/14561858.CD012105

[60] van der Heijden LB, Feskens EJM, Janse AJ. Maintenance interventions for overweight or obesity in children: A systematic review and meta-analysis. Obesity Reviews. 2018;**19**:798-809. DOI: 10.1111/obr.12664

[61] An R. Diet quality and physical activity in relation to childhood obesity. International Journal of Adolescent Medicine and Health. 2017;**29**(2):20150045. DOI: 10.1515/ijamh-2015-0045

[62] Alman KL, Lister NB, Garnett SPO, Gow ML, Aldwell K, Jebeile H. Dietetic management of obesity and severe obesity in children and adolescents: A scoping review of guidelines. Obesity Reviews. 2021;**22**:e13132. DOI: 10.1111/obr.13132

[63] Okada C, Tabuchi T, Iso H. Association between skipping breakfast in parents and children and childhood overweight/obesity among children: A nationwide 10.5-year prospective study in Japan. International Journal of Obesity (Lond). 2018;**42**:1724-1732. DOI: 10.1038/s41366-018-0066-5

[64] Karatzi K, Moschonis G, Choupi E, Manios Y, Healthy Growth Study group. Late-night overeating is associated with smaller breakfast, breakfast skipping, and obesity in children: The healthy growth study. Nutrition. 2017;**33**:141-144. DOI: 10.1016/j.nut.2016.05.010

[65] Bell S, Yew SSY, Devenish G, Ha D, Do L, Scott J. Duration of breastfeeding, but not timing of solid food, reduces the risk of overweight and obesity in children aged 24 to 36 months: Findings from an Australian cohort study. International Journal of Environmental Research and

Public Health. 2018;**15**:599. DOI: 10.3390/ijerph15040599

[66] Wang W, Wu Y, Zhang D. Association of dairy products consumption with risk of obesity in children and adults: A meta-analysis of mainly cross-sectional studies. Annals of Epidemiology. 2016;**26**:870-882.e2. DOI: 10.1016/j.annepidem.2016.09.005

[67] Pérez-Bravo F, Duarte L, Arredondo-Olguín M, Iniguez G, Castillo-Valenzuela O. Vitamin D status and obesity in children from Chile. European Journal of Clinical Nutrition. 2022;**76**:899-901. DOI: 10.1038/s41430-021-01043-9

[68] Cunha KA, Magalhaes EI, Loureiro LM, Sant'Ana LF, Ribeiro AQ, Novaes JF. Calcium intake, serum vitamin D and obesity in children: Is there an association? Revista Paulista de Pediatria. 2015;**33**:222-229. DOI: 10.1016/j.rpped.2015.03.001

[69] Altman M, Wilfley DE. Evidence update on the treatment of overweight and obesity in children and adolescents. Journal of Clinical Child and Adolescent Psychology. 2015;**44**:521-537. DOI: 10.1080/15374416.2014.963854

[70] Coles N, Birken C, Hamilton J. Emerging treatments for severe obesity in children and adolescents. BMJ. 2016;**354**:i4116. DOI: 10.1136/bmj.i4116

[71] Czepiel KS, Perez NP, Campoverde Reyes KJ, Sabharwal S, Stanford FC. Pharmacotherapy for the treatment of overweight and obesity in children, adolescents and young adults in a large health system in the US. Frontiers in Endocrinology (Lausanne). 2020;**11**:290. DOI: 10.3389/fendo.2020.00290

[72] Mead E, Atkinson G, Richter B, Metzendorf MI, Baur L, Finer N, et al. Drug interventions for the treatment of obesity in children and adolescents. Cochrane Database of Systematic Reviews. 2016;**11**:CD012436. DOI: 10.1002/14651858.CD012436

[73] Styne DM, Arslanian SA, Connor EL, Farooqi IS, Murad MH, Silverstein JH, et al. Pediatric obesity-assessment, treatment and prevention: An Endocrine Society clinical practice guideline. The Journal of Clinical Endocrinology and Metabolism. 2017;**102**:709-757. DOI: 10.1210/js.2016-2573

[74] Sherafat-Kazemzadeh R, Yanovski SZ, Yanovski JA. Pharmacotherapy for childhood obesity: Present and future prospects. International Journal of Obesity. 2013;**37**:1-15. DOI: 10.1038/ijo.2012.144

[75] Pratt JSA, Browne A, Browne NT, Bruzoni M, Cohen M, Desai A, et al. ASMBS pediatric metabolic and bariatric surgery guidelines. Surgery for Obesity and Related Diseases. 2018;**14**:882-901. DOI: 10.1016/j.soard.2018.03.019

[76] Camilleri M, Staiano A. Insights on obesity in children and adults: Individualizing management. Trends in Endocrinology and Metabolism. 2019;**30**:724-734. DOI: 10.1016/j.tem.2019.07.016

[77] Mado FG, Sirajuddin S, Muis M, Maria IL, Darmawansyah D, Arifin MA. Intervention empowerment of families in preventing and controlling overweight and obesity in children: A systematic review. Journal of Public Health Research. 2021;**10**:2185. DOI: 10.4081/jphr.2021.2185

[78] Loveman E, Al-Khudairy L, Johnson RE, Robertson W, Colquitt JL, Mead EL, et al. Parent-only interventions for childhood overweight or obesity in children aged 5 to 11 years.

Cochrane Database of Systematic Reviews. 2015;**2015**:CD012008. DOI: 10.1002/14651858.CD012008

[79] Kaur J, Lamb MM, Ogden CL. The association between food insecurity and obesity in children - the National Health and nutrition examination survey. Journal of the Academy of Nutrition and Dietetics. 2015;**115**:751-758. DOI: 10.1016/j.jand.2015.01.003

[80] Alberdi G, McNamara AE, Lindsay KL, Scully HA, Horan MH, Gibney ER, et al. The association between childcare and risk of childhood overweight and obesity in children aged 5 years and under a systematic review. European Journal of Pediatrics. 2016;**175**:1277-1294. DOI: 10.1007/s00431-016-2768-9

Chapter 2

Stigmatization of the Patients Who Live with Overweight or Obesity

Daria Lahoda

Abstract

Historically, obesity was defined by a body mass index (BMI) ≥ 30 kg/m^2. Although increased body fat can have important health and well-being implications, its presence alone does not necessarily mean or reliably predict poorer health. Overweight is defined in the case of BMI from 25 to 29.9 kg/m^2. There is a need to address this condition, as it precedes the development of obesity and requires medical intervention. Patients living with overweight or obesity often experience prejudice or stigmatization by society and/or health professionals. Weight stigmatization is a prejudiced attitude and/or discrimination against people based on a person's body weight and size. According to research, from 20 to 40% of patients living with overweight or obesity experience this attitude during their lifetime. In this study, we aimed to assess the degree of obesity and the prevalence of stigmatization among overweight and obese Ukrainians, using a questionnaire-based method.

Keywords: obesity, patient, stigmatization, overweight, bodyweight management

1. Introduction

This is a hardship that obese people encounter in various spheres of life, namely during education, employment, and when visiting medical institutions [1–4]. Often, doctors have a stereotypical mindset about patients living with overweight or obesity, who are often get described as, lacking self-control and willpower, do not follow prescribed recommendations, do not have a low level of intelligence and, in the end, it is their own fault, that they have high blood pressure or obesity [5, 6].

According to the data given in the studies, patients who are overweight or obese receive shorter consultations with doctors and doctors have less respect for such patients [7, 8]. These factors affect the quality of medical care provided to such patients and their compliance with the doctor. Doctors and nurses tend to stigmatize such patients, which is manifested in excessive attribution of medical symptoms and problems solely because the patient has increase in body weight (BW), which in turn affects diagnostic and treatment measures for such a patient [9].

Preconceptions about BW in healthcare settings may reduce the quality of care for patients living with obesity. A key factor in reducing bias, stigmatization, and discrimination in healthcare facilities is staff awareness of their own attitudes and behaviors toward people living with obesity.

Primary care clinicians should promote a holistic approach to BW and health with an emphasis on behavioral characteristics in all patients, focusing on healthy lifestyles and the underlying causes of increased BW, but avoiding stigmatization and overly simplistic statements such as "eat less and move more" [1].

It is imperative to investigate the prevalence of weight stigma in different healthcare systems, to determine the extent, nature, and factors associated with this phenomenon, and to implement interventions to eradicate and prevent it.

According to the data of the STEPS international study, which included 7,700 adults aged 18 to 69, in 2019 a quarter of the population in Ukraine was obese (BMI $\geq$30 kg/m^2), and more than 50% were overweight (BMI 25–29.9 kg/m^2) [10].

Therefore, more than half of Ukrainians currently have one or another manifestation of excess BW and may be subject to stigma regarding BW.

2. Research materials and methods

The study included 251 patients with BMI $\leq$ 25 kg/m^2 aged 18 years and older who participated in the study. The study was questionnaire-based and conducted at the Department of Family Medicine and Polyclinic Therapy of Odesa National Medical University. Patients were included in the study after completing the informed consent process, which provided an explanation of the purpose and content of the survey, as well as the names of the investigators. Potential participants were informed that the survey was anonymous, took approximately 5–10 min to complete, and that completion of the survey was optional. In addition, the respondents were informed that the results of the questionnaire will be summarized and published in the form of a scientific article. Informed consent was ensured by instructing patients to complete the questionnaire only if they agreed to participate in the survey.

The questionnaire consisted of two parts. The first included data on the age, sex, body weight, and height of the patient for further calculation of the body mass index. The second part included six open-ended questions about the characteristics of communication of a patient living with overweight or obesity with medical professionals (**Table 1**).

For clearer processing of open questions, we categorized the answers, as 0—never, 1—very rarely, 2—occasionally, 3—sometimes, 4—often, 5—always.

1 Did you feel disrespected by medical professionals because of being overweight or obesity?
2 Did you feel that your body weight prevents medical workers from providing you with medical assistance?
3 Did you feel that you received less than optimal treatment because of your body weight?
4 Did you feel judged by the medical staff because of your body weight?
5 Have there been cases when medical devices did not fit you because of your body weight?
6 Have you refused a visit to a medical institution because of a premonition that the medical staff would treat you with disdain or condemnation because of your body weight?

Table 1.
Survey question.

Answers to the survey were recorded automatically using Google forms. Surveys were conducted during 2021–2022. After the survey was completed, the data were downloaded and permanently deleted from Google Forms.

The study was performed taking into account all standards of good clinical practice and the requirements of the Declaration of Helsinki of the World Medical Association "Ethical principles of medical research with the participation of a person as a research object."

Statistical processing of the research results was carried out according to generally accepted methods of variational statistics. Reliability was assessed by student's t-test. Differences were considered significant at $p \leq 0.05$. The correlation was assessed using Spearman's correlation test and Pearson's correlation-regression analysis.

3. Research results

According to the design, our study included 251 patients whose mean age was 35.26 ± 5.27 years. There are more women among them, namely 173 women (68.92%) and 78 men (31.08%). Based on the weight and height of the patient, the BMI was determined and we were able to divide the patients according to the degree of obesity and obtained the data shown in **Table 2**.

It can be seen from **Table 2** that most of the interviewed patients had obesity class 2 (28.48%), and the fewest patients had overweight (21.12%).

When passing the second block of the survey, we had the data presented in Figure.

Figure 1 shows that the majority of patients when answering the question chose the answers "3" and "4," which are "sometimes" and "often," respectively. Let us analyze this in more detail. Thus, we received the most "never" answers to the question "Have there been cases when medical devices did not fit you because of your body weight?," namely 94 patients (37.45%). The item "very rarely" was most marked by patients in response to the question "Did you feel that you received less optimal treatment because of your body weight?," namely 74 (29, 48%) respondents.

The answer to the question "occasionally" was provided by 23.37% of patients. Participants who most often felt stigmatization expressed it in response to the question "Did you feel judged by the medical staff because of your body weight?" and "Have you refused a visit to a medical institution because of a premonition that the medical staff would treat you with disdain or judgment, because of your body weight?,": namely 41.83% and 46.61%, respectively.

The degree of obesity	Mean BMI, kg/m^2 number of patients, abs. number	Mean BMI, kg/m^2 number of patients, abs. number
Overweight	27.01 ± 0.86	53 (21.12%)
Obesity class 1	32.14 ± 1.02	68 (27.09%)
Obesity class 2	37.24 ± 0.46	74 (28.48%)
Obesity class 3	41.05 ± 1.46	56 (22.3%)

Table 2.
Distribution of patients according to the severity of obesity.

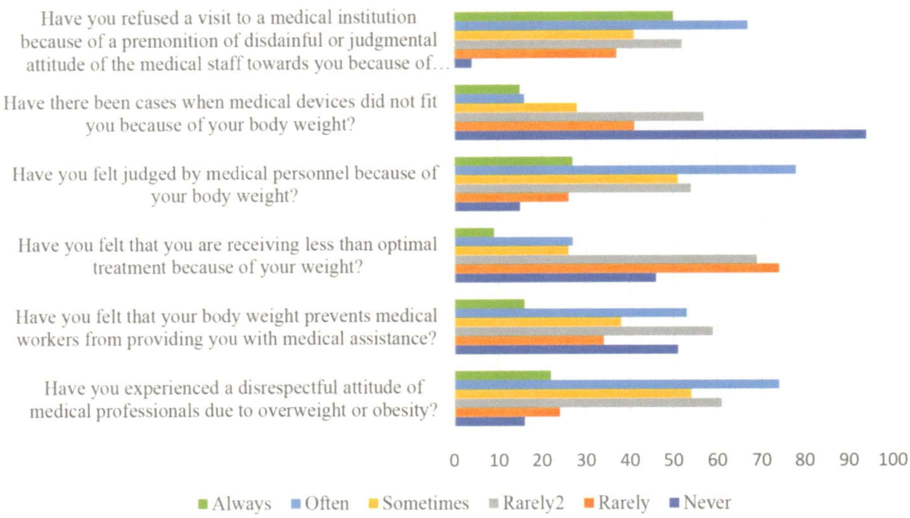

Figure 1.
Results of the second part of the survey.

At the same time, it was established that positive answers to the questions were correlated with BMI, so a direct close correlation between BMI and the feeling of stigmatization of patients was determined, namely $r = 0.81$, $p < 0.05$.

4. Discussion

The results of the survey show that the majority of patients who are overweight or obese often experience disrespect due to their overweight. In addition, the vast majority of respondents said that they avoided visits to the doctor because of the premonition that the medical staff would treat them with disdain or judgment because of their body weight. However, it must be remembered that one of the main limitations of a voluntary online survey is selection bias, that is, a greater need to answer questionnaire questions for respondents who have experienced disrespect in the past.

Thus, the rates of adverse experiences reported in our study may be higher than in the general population of people living with hyperlipidemia or obesity. Nevertheless, our results are consistent with previous studies examining the prevalence of patient stigmatization within the healthcare system [11–13]. In one study, which was also conducted on the basis of a questionnaire, 89% of patients reported that they felt inappropriate comments from doctors about their body weight [14]. In addition, in a survey of 329 health professionals who specialized in eating disorders, 56% of respondents reported that their colleagues stigmatized patients with obesity [15].

Stigma from BW can manifest itself in a variety of ways, including less patient-centeredness, a less respectful approach, less positive communication and information provision, and less time allocated to medical appointments [6]. According to studies [4, 16], a disrespectful approach is registered at various levels of medical care. The main medical professionals who were accused of negligent care were family doctors, gynecologists, traumatologists, and anesthesiologists (mainly during the administration of epidural anesthesia). Thus, these healthcare providers should be aware of the adverse impact of stigma on BW management and take a particularly sensitive approach to patients living with overweight or obesity.

5. Conclusions

When managing patients living with obesity, it is necessary to be more empathetic and sensitive. Stigmatization of this category of patients negatively affects weight loss as well as BW control. In addition, the stigmatization of a patient based on body weight affects all areas of the patient's life and, most of all, the quality of the patient's medical care. The problem of stigmatization of patients who live with overweight or obesity is relevant in Ukraine. But currently, we do not have enough such data on Ukrainians. The medical community should be aware of the existence of the problem of stigmatization of the patient according to body weight and also introduce mechanisms to overcome this problem.

Author details

Daria Lahoda
Philosophy in Medicine, Department of Family Medicine and Polyclinic Therapy, Odesa National Medical University, Odesa, Ukraine

*Address all correspondence to: dlagoda19@gmail.com

References

[1] CMAJ. Canada Obesity in Adults: A Clinical Practice Guideline. Available from: https://www.cmaj.ca/content/192/31/E875

[2] Mulherin K, Miller YD, Barlow FK, Diedrichs PC, Thompson R. Weight stigma in maternity care: Women's experiences and care providers' attitudes. BMC Pregnancy and Childbirth. 2013;**13**:19

[3] Spahlholz J, Baer N, Konig HH, Riedel-Heller SG, Luck-Sikorski C. Obesity and discrimination—A systematic review and meta-analysis of observational studies. Obesity Reviews. 2016;**17**(1):43-55

[4] Puhl RM, Heuer CA. The stigma of obesity: A review and update. Obesity (Silver Spring). 2009;**17**(5):941-964

[5] Rubino F, Puhl RM, Cummings DE, Eckel RH, Ryan DH, Mechanick JI, et al. Joint international consensus statement for ending stigma of obesity. Nature Medicine. 2020;**26**(4):485-497

[6] Phelan SM, Burgess DJ, Yeazel MW, Hellerstedt WL, Griffin JM, van Ryn M. Impact of weight bias and stigma on quality of care and outcomes for patients with obesity. Obesity Reviews. 2015;**16**(4):319-326

[7] Huizinga MM, Cooper LA, Bleich SN, Clark JM, Beach MC. Physician respect for patients with obesity. Journal of General Internal Medicine. 2009;**24**(11):1236-1239

[8] Hebl MR, Xu J. Weighing the care: Physicians' reactions to the size of a patient. International Journal of Obesity and Related Metabolic Disorders. 2001;**25**(8):1246-1252

[9] Persky S, Eccleston CP. Medical student bias and care recommendations for an obese versus non-obese virtual patient. International Journal of Obesity. 2011;**35**(5):728-735

[10] World Health Organization. Available from: https://apps.who.int/iris/bitstream/handle/10665/336643/WHO-EURO-2020-1468-41218-56059-ukr.pdf?sequence=1&isAllowed=y [Accessed: May 15, 2023]

[11] Remmert JE, Convertino AD, Roberts SR, Godfrey KM, Butryn ML. Stigmatizing weight experiences in health care: Associations with BMI and eating behaviours. Obesity Science and Practice. 2019;**5**(6):555-563

[12] Tomiyama AJ, Carr D, Granberg EM, Major B, Robinson E, Sutin AR, et al. How and why weight stigma drives the obesity "epidemic" and harms health. BMC Medicine. 2018;**16**(1):123

[13] Schwartz MB, Chambliss HO, Brownell KD, Blair SN, Billington C. Weight bias among health professionals specializing in obesity. Obesity Research. 2003;**11**(9):1033-1039

[14] Friedman KE, Reichmann SK, Costanzo PR, Zelli A, Ashmore JA, Musante GJ. Weight stigmatization and ideological beliefs: Relation to psychological functioning in obese adults. Obesity Research. 2005;**13**(5):907-916

[15] Puhl RM, Latner JD, King KM, Luedicke J. Weight bias among professionals treating eating disorders: Attitudes about treatment and perceived patient outcomes. The International Journal of Eating Disorders. 2014;**47**(1):65-75

[16] Puhl RM, Heuer CA. Obesity stigma: Important considerations for public health. American Journal of Public Health. 2010;**100**(6):1019-1028

Section 2

Metabolic and Neurogenic Effects of Obesity: Implications for Chronic Diseases

Chapter 3

Metabolic Changes in Obesity

Maritza Torres Valdez and Valmore José Bermúdez Pirela

Abstract

The exact basis for the increase in global obesity rates is complex, so obesity should not be simply viewed as a biochemical problem of energy imbalance. While imbalance in energy metabolism is the main cause of obesity, only 5% of patients return to a normal weight after the incorporation of dietary changes. Eating behavior is enormously complex. It is governed by brain biochemistry influenced by many interdependent peptides or lipids. Excess body fat is the defining characteristic of this disorder, linked to the occurrence of a number of metabolic irregularities, which lead to other health problems. Adipose tissue plays an essential role in the metabolic process of energy balance, essential for understanding the phenomena associated with obesity.

Keywords: metabolism, obesity, food, energy, biochemistry

1. Introduction

1.1 Definition of obesity

Obesity has been defined and categorized by the application of body mass index (BMI), the most used indirect method to define and classify it, which is limited by its low specificity of 36–66% because this method does not allow to distinguish adipose tissue, as well as hydration index or fat mass. However, it continues to be widely used in all age groups because it is simple to apply and economic [1].

Pasca and Montero take a different approach [1]. They did not define obesity as an increase in adipose tissue, but evaluated it as a systemic pathology where various organs are involved, resulting in a deterioration of metabolism, characterized by inflammatory processes, expressed according to the relationship between the genome and the environment, where the phenotypic expression is acquired as a product of this interaction, mainly the increased deposition of adipose tissue [1].

1.2 Ubiquity of adipose tissue

Adipose tissue constitutes 20–28% of the weight in healthy people and 80% in obese people, depending on several factors such as sex, energy status, distribution, and location of adipose tissue that affect its function [2].

Preadipocytes, adipocytes, fibroblasts, macrophages, monocytes, vascular stromal cells, and innervating cells are among the variety of cell types seen in adipose tissue; however, most of these cells do not appear to be adipocytes [3]. Up to 80% of the DNA obtained from adipose tissue is derived from vascular cell, fibroblast, leukocyte, and macrophage; three varieties of adipose tissue coexist according to function, color, vascularization, and structure [4].

As part of the connective tissue group, adipose tissue provides cohesion to organs or systems, supports structure, and is a key regulator of energy balance [5]. It is a complex endocrine tissue with high metabolic activity, and its function is to maintain energy balance, manage body temperature, regulate lipid and glucose metabolism, control blood pressure, and prevent blood clotting processes [6, 7].

Obese persons produce less elastin and more collagen types I, III, V, and VI, bronectin, and laminin in their adipose tissue than lean people [8]. These changes promote the growth of fibrotic tissue, which is more common in visceral fat than in subcutaneous fat [8]. Fibrosis, which favors lipid storage in the liver, pancreas, heart, skeletal muscle, limits the process of adipose tissue expansion. Collectively, these changes lead to lipotoxicity [8, 9].

Hepatic overload caused by fatty acid accumulation is the origin of increased hepatic gluconeogenesis and lipoprotein metabolism in hepatocytes, which also prevent the breakdown of insulin and apolipoprotein B [8, 9].

2. Types of adipose tissue

2.1 White adipose tissue

In each adipose cell of the target tissue there is a lipid vacuole, where lipids are stored for use when energy demand is required [10]. Triacylglycerols make up 90–99% of the total lipids in the vacuole and provide sufficient energy to meet the daily energy needs of an adult [10, 11].

White adipose tissue produces proteins with a wide range of functions in relation to immunity, proinflammatory cytokines, complement, fibrinolytic system, renin–angiotensin system, lipid mobilization, and steroid enzymes. It also produces large amounts of adipokines and lipokines, which act as metabolic regulatory hormones [2].

Table 1 demonstrates the correlation between adipokines or lipokines produced with anti-inflammatory activity and those with pro-inflammatory and proatherogenic action in metabolic variations in obesity [12].

When there is an excess of energy, the functionality of adipocytes decreases, which is reflected in the imbalance of adipokine production [12]. Adipose tissue can buffer energy profusion through lipid storage is the result of proper expansion of this tissue, which is a sign of proper functionality [13].

Adipose tissue can develop through hyperplasia and hypertrophy and degenerate into malfunction with excess energy. This results in cardiometabolic risk leading to increased lipid deposition and decreased lipid utilization [5, 13].

2.2 Adipocytes

They are considered specialized cells that store lipids, but this is not their primary purpose, as evidenced by beta cells, muscle cells, and neurons [14]. Mature adipocytes develop when markers include the expression and adipocyte-associated hormones, cytokines, and enzymes associated with lipid storage and release into the bloodstream [14].

Adipokine/lipokine	Metabolic effect	Secretory organ or tissue
Leptin	Thermogenesis, lipid oxidation, insulin sensitivity, and anorexigenic impact.	Adipocytes, epithelium of the stomach and intestines, placenta, muscles, mammary gland, and brain.
Adiponectin	Lipid oxidation, reduction of liver gluconeogenesis, reduction of monocyte adhesion, reduction of inflammation and atherosclerotic risk, and anorexigenic effects.	Adipocytes
Omentin	Increased glucose uptake prompted by insulin and peptide release of orexigenic peptides are two aspects of orexigenic impact.	Intestinal cells, vascular stroma, and visceral adipose tissue.
Resistin	Insulin resistance and fatty acid synthesis in the liver have anorectic effects.	Adipocytes
Reintol-4 binding protein	Altered GLUT4 expression leads to reduced retinol transport and insulin resistance.	Adipocytes
Quemerin	If administered persistently, it causes adipogenesis, angiogenesis, proinflammatory, and orexigenic effects.	Adipocytes, hepatocytes, and lung cells
Vistatin	Proinflammatory and proatherogenic factor affecting the development of obesity.	Visceral adipocytes
Palmitoleic acid	Lipogenesis is decreased by insulin.	Adipocytes
Palmitic acid-hydroxyl-stearic acid (PAHSA)	The synthesis of insulin, glucagon-like peptide 1 and other hormones, glucose uptake and anti- inflammatory actions.	Fasting subcutaneous and peri-gonadal adipocytes.

Table 1.
Adipokines/lipokines, metabolic effect, and secretory organ or tissue.

Perhaps the most interesting aspect of adipocyte differentiation is the way in which preadipocytes are added to the adipocyte repertoire, a repertoire of peroxisome-activated receptor family members and protein receptors that bind CCAAT enhancers [14].

Mature adipocytes are highly specialized cells that are central to energy storage and delivery mechanisms and are subject to very tight central and peripheral control, given these characteristics, it is not uncommon to find that adipose tissue is part of several axes, such as the adipose–insulin axis, the adipocyte–vascular–brain axis, and the adipocyte–myocyte axis [14, 15].

On another scale, the metabolic activity of adipocytes changes significantly in the hypoxia state. Indeed, some glycolytic enzyme genes, such as hexokinase 2 (HK2), phosphofructokinase (PFKP), and GLUT1, show increased expression in cultured adipocyte cells under hypoxia conditions. Moreover, while GLUT4 is the predominant isoform in adipocytes, GLUT1 is the most efficient glucose transporter at low oxygen levels. These changes suggest that adipocytes have increased glucose uptake and metabolism, as expected in hypoxic areas, which are supported by their increased secretion of lactate [15].

2.3 Myocytes

Myocytes are affected by obesity, while adipocytes slowly perish from asphyxia [15, 16]. The adipo–hypoglycemic axis plays a key role in obesity and accompanying diseases, such as type 2 diabetes, due to their mutual interaction. Under conditions of overfeeding, adipose tissue does not store excess energy in an adequate manner, resulting in a "spillover" impact on the entire body [15, 16].

2.4 Adiponectin

Adiponectin normalizes glucose metabolism and enables regulation of vascular homeostasis by interfering with key signaling pathways in the endothelial cells and reducing inflammatory activity in the subendothelial region. Adiponectin levels are often low in obese individuals, indicating that obesity, diabetes mellitus type 2 (DM2), and cardiovascular disease (CVD) are examples of insulin-resistant and inflammatory conditions that reduce the amount of insulin produced [17, 18].

Two receptors, AdipoR1 and AdipoR2, were initially cloned in 2003 by Yamauchi et al., modulate the actions of adiponectin [16]. Like the G protein-coupled-receptor (GPCRs) group, being an integral membrane protein with seven transmembrane domains. Adiponectin receptors, unlike GPCRs, have an internal N-terminal and an external C-terminal domain, both receptor subtypes can form homo- and heteromultinomers [18, 19]. In the pancreatic cell, high amounts of fatty acids (FAs) enhance the production of lipoprotein lipase, both receptors have been identified [18, 19].

2.5 Brown or brown adipose tissue (BAT)

This tissue in humans has metabolically active structures, and it consumes energy through thermogenesis to regulate body temperature [12]. It regulates energy balance by regulating metabolism. This is done by stimulating uncoupling proteins, and it uses proton flux from oxidative phosphorylation to produce heat, by activating beta-adrenergic receptors in this tissue [20].

The brown adipocyte is a biological heat-producing powerhouse due to its unique ability to uncouple the process of oxidative phosphorylation and respiratory chain in its mitochondria [21]. As of the uncoupling protein UCP1, which renders the inner membrane of mitochondria proton permeable and causes brown adipocyte mitochondria to act as a metabolic substrate oxidation machine to produce heat rather than AT, this tissue is active in adults and abnormally inactive in obese people [21].

Differentiation in certain brown adipose tissue areas of white adipose cells, and increased activation of adrenaline and some cytokines promote trans-adaptive thermogenesis. This increases the expression of UCP1, the presence of brown and beige adipose tissue markers, enhances energy consumption, and promotes glucose tolerance [22]. The ability of brown and beige adipocytes to convert chemical energy into heat contributes to adaptive thermogenesis, a metabolic process whose metabolic function is correlated with a person's overall metabolic profile [22].

2.6 Beige adipose tissue

When experimental animals were exposed to prolonged cold to induce thermogenesis, beige adipose tissue (BAT) activation occurred with the development of brown adipose tissue at sites typical of white adipose tissue [23, 24].

Beige adipocytes that develop at the level of white adipose tissue have a completely different cell lineage than "traditional" brown adipocytes, according to several studies [25, 26].

Investigation of the browning process as a means of promoting BAT activity in the organism is of interest given this, along with the inducibility in the development of beige adipocytes in response to environmental variables [23, 24].

Following transdifferentiation, UCP1-expressing beige adipocytes can manifest in response to hormones, exercise, or cold exposure. These cells show a pattern of thermal gene expression that elevates energy and oxygen consumption [27]. Adipose tissue depots wait for environmental cues to become active, activating hormones such as leptin, FGF 21, and U2P (UF2) [3].

3. Vasocrine regulation in pathological conditions

Consistent with the plasticity of adipocytes observed in their preadipocyte differentiation into macrophages and hypertrophy/hyperplasia of differentiated adipocytes, the epicardial adipocyte also undergoes several changes [25]. Elevated synthesis of saturated free FAs, which bind toll-like receptor-4 (TLR-4) in macrophages and activate NF-kB, as well as increased TNF-α, are two modifications observed in larger adipocytes [25, 26]. However, macrophages may also develop from monocytes that spread through the subendothelial region via CAM-1 and MCP-1, rather than solely from differentiated preadipocytes [25, 26].

Most of the adipokines generated from adipose tissues have receptors expressed on blood arteries, which is crucial for cardiovascular pathology [28]. Proinflammatory adipokines are transported from epicardial fat to the vascular wall much more easily and efficiently due to the proximity of the epicardial adipose tissue (EAT) and coronary arteries. TNF from EAT readily diffuses into the blood arteries during RV by blocking the PI3K pathway in the endothelial cells [28].

In situations of insulin resistance, it has been confirmed that increased TNF-α locally induces a vasoconstriction related to ET-1 synthesis in coronary artery endothelium [25]. Together with the maintenance of chronic inflammation and insulin resistance in endothelial cells, this also plays a role. The extracellular signal-regulated kinase, which moves from the cytosol to the nucleus and triggers ET-1 production, is phosphorylated in this TNF-activated pathway [26, 28].

4. Energy metabolism of obesity

Imbalances in energy metabolism can lead to obesity [29]. In general, molecules that cause hunger tend to reduce energy expenditure, and compounds that cause satiety tend to increase the body's energy expenditure. This is because the basic mechanism of biochemical control of energy behavior is highly redundant and pleiotropic. This is congruent with the energy saving or energy expenditure tactics that the body uses depending on physiological and dietary circumstances [29].

According to Rial-Pensado et al. [30], the AMP-activated kinase enzyme plays a crucial role in this process by regulating brain-derived signals that regulate energy balance from the hypothalamus [30].

The malfunctioning of both cell typologies is due to an increase in white fat cells and a reduction in brown fat cells as a result of excessive energy intake [31]. The intervention of the immune system in adipocytes is crucial to maintain the balance in both tissues and favors the oxidation of FAs, which prevail in brown and beige cells [31].

It is important to understand these connections and the sequence of events that occur throughout the development of obesity [32].

4.1 Obesity and energy balance

The energy balance is neutral when these two variables are equal, i.e. balance between intake and expenditure; when there is an imbalance if the energy intake is greater than that expended, as with obesity, body weight slowly increases [33].

At the biochemical and physiological level, the many components of the energy balance equation are intrinsically related, so that alterations in one component of the equation may have a reverse effect on another; conversely, when food is restricted, as in the case of fasting, energy is conserved, and appetite is increased [33]. Despite these homeostatic reactions to preserve homeostasis, sedentary habits and/or chronic caloric excess can affect the efficacy of these regulatory mechanisms [33].

4.2 Hypothalamic regulation of energy balance

The hypothalamus is divided into nuclei or clusters of anatomically distinct neurons, which are linked by axonal projections to form neural circuits. The neuropeptides orexigenic, feeding promoter, agouti-related protein (AgRP), and neuropeptide Y are expressed by a cluster of neurons [34]. A second population of neurons expresses the anorexigenic products propiomelanocortin, which is the precursor of melanocyte alpha-stimulating hormone; these neurons project to other second-order neurons present in other hypothalamic nuclei [33].

The dorsomedial, lateral, and paraventricular nuclei are some of the secondary hypothalamic nuclei served by this group of first-order neurons, which send their axons widely to the central nervous system (CNS) [34]. The ventromedial nucleus of the hypothalamus, which is dorsal to the arcuate nucleus (ARC), receives mainly projections from AgRP/NPY and CART/POMC neurons. Axons from ventromedial nucleus (VMH) neurons also travel to the ARC, secondary hypothalamic nuclei, and brainstem areas [34].

4.3 AMPK

In eukaryotes, an enzyme known as an AMP-driven protein kinase functions as an energy sensor [35]. AMP-activated protein kinase (AMPK) is a heterotrimeric complex that exists at the molecular level. It consists of two regulatory and catalytic subunits that include serine/threonine protein kinase domains that are phosphorylated at threonine. The AMPK complex can exist in 12 different configurations in mammals because several genes are involved in the expression of each component [36].

4.4 Hypothalamic AMPK as a regulator of ingestion

ARC, paraventricular nucleus (PVN), VMH, and lateral hypothalamic area (LHA) are some of the hypothalamic areas where AMPK is expressed. The fact that AMPK modification is associated with insulin resistance, obesity, hormonal problems, metabolic changes, and cardiovascular disease serves as evidence of its physiological value [36].

Accordingly, fasting elevates hypothalamic AMPK activity, while refeeding inhibits it, acting as an energy sensor [37]. There is evidence linking hypothalamic

AMPK in the regulation of food intake. The orexigenic function of ghrelin is related to several findings on the hypothalamic role of AMPK in the management of energy balance [36].

4.5 Hypothalamic AMPK as a regulator of thermogenesis

Hypothalamic AMPK is involved in the control of brown adipose tissue thermogenesis by the CNS. Pharmacological and genetic studies demonstrate that VMH causes a decrease in weight and increase in the thermogenic program in the BAT in depletion of AMPK, the deduction of its activity, in response to thyroid hormones increases thermogenesis [34, 37].

4.6 A regulator of glucose homeostasis: Hypothalamic AMPK

These neurons are found in specific regions of the brain, including certain hypothalamic nuclei. Excess glucose inhibits the ability of the hypothalamus to activate AMPK, resulting in prolonged hypoglycemia. The ARC and VMH primarily control this impact. By fusing nutritional and hormonal information in the hypothalamus, AMPK functions as a crucial sensor in energy balance [36].

By accumulating altered lipid species that are "toxic," lipotoxicity affects cellular functioning as well as organs and tissues. Most of these lipid species have critical structural, signaling, or bioenergetic substrate functions that support the equilibrium state of the cell. However, harmful lipid derivatives can be produced by lipid species that are created as a direct result of chemical agents of reactive oxygen or nitrogen agents [36].

4.7 Pathophysiological and metabolic changes in obesity

Lipid reserve, prolonged inflammation, tissue hypoxia, endoplasmic reticulum (ER) stress **(Figure 1)**, and the emergence of insulin resistance constitute the physiological process of the development of overweight to obesity [38].

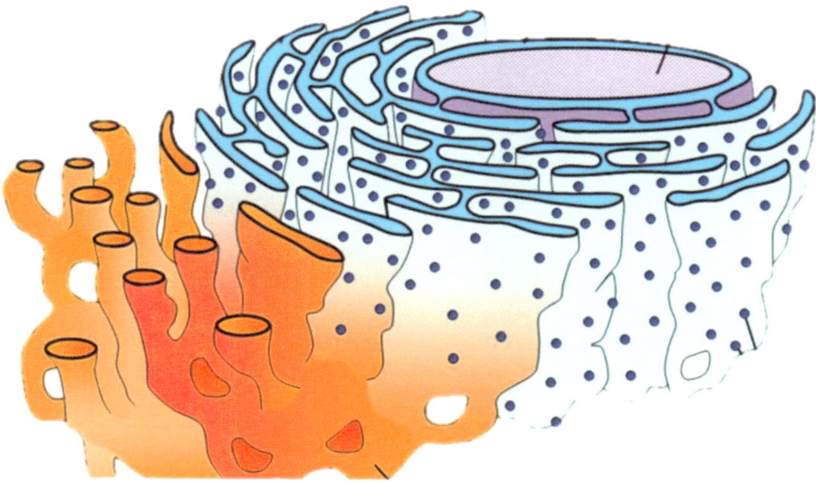

Figure 1.
The endoplasmic reticulum (ER) is a central cell organelle in which transmembrane and secretory proteins are synthesized, folded and matured.

The ER is a central cell organelle in which transmembrane and secretory proteins are synthesized, folded, and matured.

4.8 Lipid accumulation

Increased visceral and intra-abdominal fat is a sign of systemic fat deposition which triggers the production of cytokines that favor the onset of insulin resistance, inflammation, and development of cardiovascular pathology [31, 39].

5. Lipoinflammation in obesity

Adipose tissue has a significant impact on the inflammatory, antifibrinolytic, and vasoactive cascades, indicating that it has an immediate effect on the inflammatory process [38, 40]. Adipocytokines, which are elevated by hyperplasia, proliferation, and differentiation of preadipocytes, are the cytokines responsible for controlling the physiological response of adipose tissues [40].

The visceral fat depot expands with decreasing lipogenic capacity and by the process of hypertrophy, when the subcutaneous adipose tissue does not adequately store surplus energy exceeding the storage level [41].

The release of proinflammatory adipocytokines causes the macrophage scrolling inhibitor, IL-6 metalloproteinases, PAI-1, the vascular endothelial growth factor leptin [42]. Oxygen triggers cell death in the more peripheral fat cells, which transcribe into increased inflammation [42]. Hypoxia of adipose tissue is generated with death of peripheral adipocytes, transformation of M2 to M1 macrophages, angiogenesis, and increased production of inflammatory and anti-inflammatory proadipocytokines as shown in **(Figure 2)** [43].

This dysregulation is the result of adiponectin's disabling of NF-kB activation [43]. Macrophages located in obese adipose tissue alter and remodel with marked

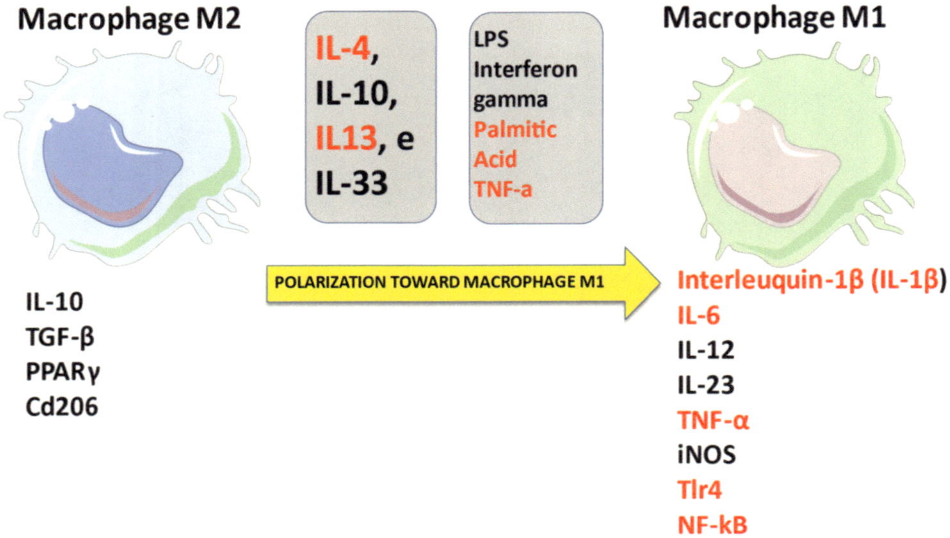

Figure 2.
Source: Valmore Bermúdez.

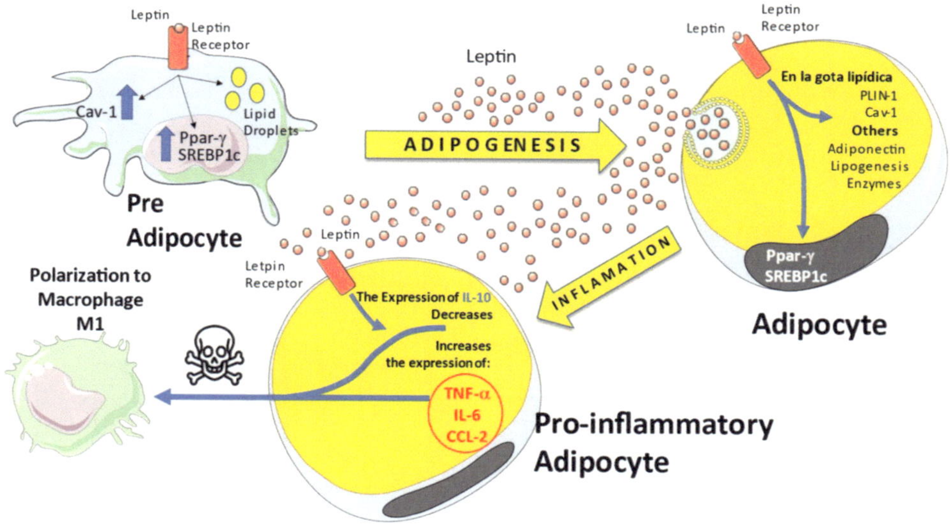

Figure 3.
Source: Valmore Bermúdez.

heterogeneity in activity and function due to complex metabolic and immunological changes that vary according to the expression of specific antigens [43].

The phenomenon of a transient "phenotypic shift" from the primarily anti-inflammatory M2 state of macrophage polarization to the more pro-inflammatory M1 form takes place during negative energy equilibrium [44].

The percentage of macrophages increased from 10–40% in the cells responsible for the release of proinflammatory chemicals, particularly TNF, in more than 50% of adipose tissue as shown in **(Figure 3)** [44, 45].

Metabolic and inflammatory processes are strongly connected and influence the progression of obesity, despite the fact that the mechanism of macrophage incorporation and adipose tissue filtration operate independently [45].

One of the most important indicators of subclinical inflammation is C-reactive protein (CRP) [46]. Regarding the regulation of macrophages, CRP has been related to M1 polarization, which is created in stimulating endothelial cells to produce M-CSF and activates NF-B [47]. Finally, since adiponectin is a hormone that promotes M2 polarization through AMPK, PPAR-, and PPAR-, low levels of adiponectin, as observed in the presence of visceral obesity, also favor M1 polarization [47, 48].

M2 polarization requires the attenuation of several mediators that promote M1 [49]. In this regard, the p50 subunit of NF-B has been found to inhibit NF-B-induced M1 polarization. Similarly, the complement protein C1q has been found to inhibit NF-B activation of macrophages during endocytosis and processing of lipoproteins, reducing the release of inflammatory cytokines [47, 49, 50].

As can be seen, macrophage polarization in each situation is a power play, the outcome of which is determined by the most common type of microenvironmental stimuli as can be seen in **(Figure 4)** [47, 50].

5.1 Consequences of lipoinflammation

Lipoinflammation involves a number of interconnected pathways that support and maintain obesity [51]. Chronic acceleration of proinflammatory pathways is one of the

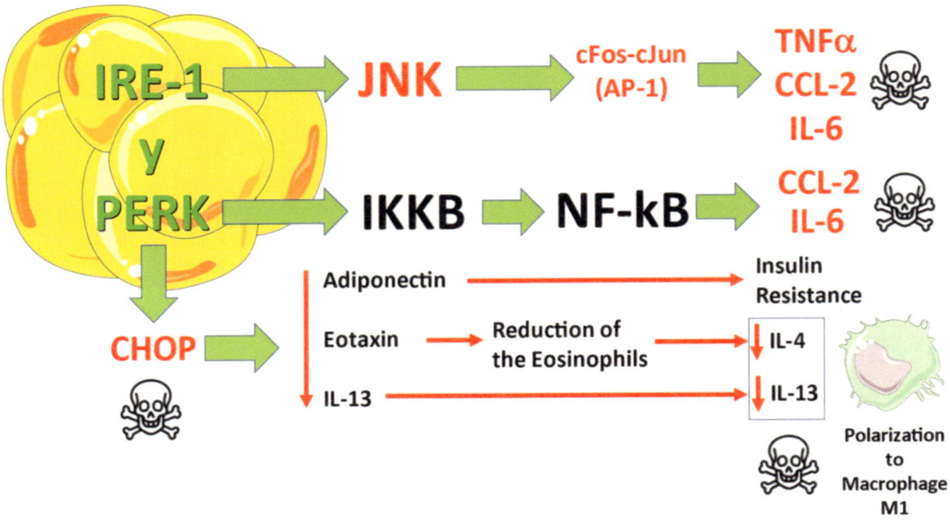

Figure 4.
Source: Valmore Bermúdez.

key processes underlying the relationship between a chronic low-grade lipoinflammatory state, the emergence of insulin resistance, and development of comorbidities [52, 53].

According to the study, comorbidities, persistent low-grade lipoinflammation, and the occurrence of insulin resistance are related [53]. The maintenance of plasma insulin levels is known as hyperinsulinemia [53].

At the level of the CNS, insulin inhibits the action of leptin, promoting satiety and energy expenditure [51, 53]. The catalytic portion of the receptor is activated by binding to its transmembrane receptor heterotetrameric [51, 53].

To bind to more intracellular substrates and maintain signaling, the receptor undergoes autophosphorylation [54]. Phosphorylated tyrosine residues bind and phosphorylate various substrate proteins of the insulin receptor, allowing phosphoinosidase to bind and become active, thus connecting insulin signaling with neuronal firing rate regulation [51].

The signal transducer and transcription generator (STAT), which links insulin signaling to gene transcription of neurotransmitters responsible for appetite control and thermogenesis, is phosphorylated following phosphorylation of JAK-2 [51].

The hormone leptin is a part of the class I cytokine receptors lacking intrinsic catalytic activity. The JAK-2 enzyme binds to the leptin receptor forming a dimeric structure when bound to it, favoring the uptake of a second adjacent receptor unit [55].

A protein called STAT-3 is also recruited and phosphorylated, and it is this protein that is ultimately responsible for sending the leptin signal to the nucleus, controlling neurotransmitter transcription [55]. The signaling molecule involved in the anorexigenic effects of leptin is STAT-3, which regulates the transcriptional activity of numerous different genes [54, 55].

When SOCS3 is increased, it interacts with the leptin-JAK-2 receptor and disables leptin signaling [56]. The JAK-2/STAT-3 pathway is predominantly regulated by leptin in the hypothalamus, and insulin modulates this pathway [54]. There is a crosstalk in the insulin and leptin signaling pathways in the regulation of the satiety mechanism [55].

5.2 Lipotoxicity due to lipid modification

Some lipids play substantial roles in revising the catalytic activity of enzymes and their cellular localization, in addition to their structural and cell signaling functions, for example, by allowing translocation to the plasma membrane or the nucleus [31]. In describing the lipid modifications that determine lipotoxicity, we can also include modifications caused by the products of lipid peroxidation. In particular, we can focus on 4-hydroxynonenal, malondialdehyde and acrolein, which can mediate lipid elimination and, at the same time, have effects other than toxicity, such as the formation of amino acid side-chain conduits [31].

5.3 Hypoxia and ER stress

Obesity generates an increase in tissue irrigation, as the amount of adipose tissue directly affects blood flow [38]. In this situation, the aforementioned pro-inflammatory systems are activated, which is considered an aggression, favoring the reduction of blood flow and thus restricting the inflow of nutrients and unregulated tissue growth [38].

Nitric oxide is an important vasodilator of adipose tissue and is produced more frequently in hypoxic environments [57]. Anaerobic glycolysis is initiated, which releases energy in the form of ATP and changes the redox state of the cell, leading to a decrease in oxygen level, maintaining tissue hypoxia, and inducing acidification [57].

It generates dysfunction of mitochondria and ER, affects the insulin signaling pathway, and favors the secretion of proinflammatory cytokines in tissue [57].

The malfunction of protein production is called ER stress, also known as ER dysfunction. Due to a deposit of defective unfolded or misfolded proteins into the lumen of the ER or excessive protein production [58]. This response is triggered by any physiological or pathological circumstance that obstructs the ability of the ER to fold proteins. Inflammation and insulin resistance associated with obesity are closely related to UPR activation [58].

Adipocyte lipolysis is mediated by ER stress, by producing more IL-6 and less leptin and adiponectin, contributes to dysregulation of adipokine secretion [57, 58].

6. Insulin resistance

The increased blood glucose level causes the pancreatic islets of Langerhans to secrete insulin, which causes these tissues to take up more glucose. In addition, hepatic and muscle glycogen generation is enhanced by the process of dephosphorylation and activation of glycogen synthase [59].

Through activation of SREBP-1c, insulin exerts a hypogenic influence on lipid metabolism, promoting lipid synthesis and reducing lipid degradation. Insulin directly affects the expression, phosphorylation, and dephosphorylation of enzymes involved in gluconeogenesis and hepatic glycogenolysis [59].

Insulin resistance inhibits the body's ability to regulate blood glucose by reducing the cellular responsiveness to normal amounts of circulating insulin [60].

The insulin-signaling pathway is regulated by the insulin receptor, a tyrosine kinase that phosphorylates receptor substrates upon binding and activation. The expression, substrate binding, phosphorylation, and kinase activity of the insulin receptor can be modified [51].

Such phosphorylation can lead to the activation of the two major protein kinase signaling pathways, the mitogen-activated protein kinases/extracellular signal-regulated kinases (MAPK/ERK) and serine–threonine Akt pathways, responsible for the arrangement of cell growth, gene expression, and protein synthesis and glucose uptake [51].

Excessive increase of lipids, triacylglycerol, saturated FAs in myocytes, promotes the synthesis of harmful lipid intermediates such as ceramides and diacylglycerols which have an adverse effect on insulin signaling, persistent inflammation, influences insulin signaling, where invading macrophages, release more TNF, thereby activating c-Jun-terminal kinase (JNK) and kappa-B kinase (IKK) signaling kinases promoting serine phosphorylation at IRS-1, favoring the onset of insulin resistance and type 2 diabetes [61].

7. Metabolic stages of obesity

In obesity, there are three metabolic stages involved in its development.

7.1 Insulin control: gradual weight gain

Insulin stimulates the production of glycogen, an energy store, and glucose oxidation at the hepatic level during the postprandial phase, producing ATP as an energy source and maintaining stable glucose levels between meals and during sleep. The liver uses a process called lipogenesis to convert the extra glucose into FAs [62, 63].

High-density lipoprotein transports the excess cholesterol to the hepatic level, where it interacts with nascent LDLV once in the blood (reverse cholesterol transport) [62, 63].

7.2 Liver and adipose tissue metabolism under insulin control

Adipose tissue: lipoprotein lipase (LPL) breaks down TGs into FAs and glycerol when mature VLDLs transport TGs into adipose tissue (the activity of this enzyme is insulin-dependent). As soon as the FAs enter the adipocytes, they are esterified with the help of glycerol phosphate, which is produced there by the glucose that was introduced by Glut-4 under the effect of insulin, then the liver receives the glycerol again [49, 51].

Adipocytes fill with TGs from the liver as they gain weight, even though the person is initially normoinsulinemic, normo-glycemic, and has normal lipid readings [49]. Depending on the level of adipose tissue storage, the duration of the "honeymoon" can vary adipogenesis, lipogenesis, apoptosis, and angiogenesis. This time span is short in people with low-lipid storage capacity; it is prolonged in those with high capacity. This process depends to a large extent on the anatomical compartment where the adipose tissue accumulates [62].

7.3 Adipose tissue storage

Adipocyte hyperplasia and adipocyte hypertrophy are inherited processes that affect the storage capacity of adipocytes [49].

7.4 Molecular factors influencing body fat distribution

Body fat distribution and total adiposity have an impact on systemic metabolism, and changes in either can increase the risk of metabolic pathology [63].

According to the amount of TG present, each anatomical depot has between 10 and 100 billion white adipocytes ranging in size from 10 to 200 microns [49]. The ability of the adipocytes in each depot to undergo hyperplasia and hypertrophy determines the amount of growth that each depot can support [49].

When the size of an adipocyte reaches a "critical" point where it can no longer expand, recruitment of preadipocytes occurs; the extent of this recruitment will depend on the pool of available adipocyte precursor cells. Adipocytes tend to evolve in both size and number over the course of growth [53, 63].

Subcutaneous adipocytes have a half-life of up to 10 years [53]. In addition to the recruitment of APCs and preadipocytes, the adipocyte undergoes continuous remodeling or turnover in which senescent and dysfunctional adipocytes are replaced by new differentiated adipocytes [53]. This continuous replacement is necessary because older adipocytes deteriorate, lose sensitivity to insulin action, and develop a proinflammatory phenotype [63].

It is believed that there are several interacting variables, which differ depending on the growth and age of the individual, resulting in epigenetic modifications that can be passed on from generation to generation, restricting the ability of adipocytes to grow and perform healthy remodeling [64].

Therefore, it can be assumed that a "metabolically ill" patient will have lower levels of APC, restricted adipocyte remodeling, less hyperplasia, and greater adipocyte hypertrophy, all leading to metabolic dysfunction [63]. On the other hand, regardless of the degree of obesity, a "metabolically healthy" obese person has more adipocyte hyperplasia in the abdominal subcutaneous depot, which is associated with metabolic health [63, 64].

8. B. Insulin control vs. counterinsulin control

When a person approaches the limit of storage capacity, they generate insulin resistance. Insulin levels are higher than physiological levels in maintaining blood glucose below 100 mg/dl, as defined by IR [63].

Adipose tissue develops insulin resistance (stage D) through upregulation of insulin receptors and increased sensitivity to hormones that act as counterinsulins (CI), including glucagon, cortisol, and adrenaline. These hormones trigger hormone sensitive lipase (HSL), an enzyme that controls the lipolytic process of TG breakdown [63].

Now that the partially filled adipocyte has room to store TG once more, insulin can activate LPL, causing it to fill with TG once more [63]. When the storage capacity of an adipocyte is exceeded, an inflammatory response is generated and the adipocyte releases cytokines that attract macrophages to the adipose tissue (stage F) [62, 63].

The TG overloaded adipocyte (stage A) undergoes morphological and functional changes and secretes resistin, infiltrating macrophages that produce TNF and other proinflammatory cytokines that permanently maintain the IR state, permanently slowing cell metabolism (stage C) [38].

Compensatory hyperinsulinemia is necessary to reverse the disabling of insulin action caused by -TNF and resistin, allowing the adipocyte to refill with TG (phase D). Plasma TG levels at this time may be normal, above the upper limit, or even only slightly above the upper limit [63].

8.1 Perpetuation of insulin resistance in adipose tissue

FAs created by lipolysis act on pancreatic beta cells, initially increasing insulin secretion. However, over time, they cause lipotoxicity by producing ceramides, which lead to cell deterioration processes by releasing cytochrome C from the mitochondria. As a result, pancreatic beta cells undergo apoptosis, which reduces insulin release. Reduced insulin secretion potentiates the influence of anti-insulin hormone, raising blood GA levels and increasing lipolysis, which affects skeletal muscle [62, 65].

GAs from hydrolysis of TGs exceed glucose from muscle glycogen storage because of palmitic acid, the fatty acid that accumulates most frequently [63, 65]. This limits the absorption of blood glucose from food and excess glycogen. Skeletal muscle glycogen stores remain full or partially full, making it difficult for the muscle to continue to absorb blood glucose from food, increasing postprandial glucose levels [66].

9. C. Contrainsulin control

TI impaired gluconeogenesis results in uncontrolled creation of glucose at the hepatic level from the amino acids created by the breakdown of protein [66]. Glucotoxicity and lipotoxicity in pancreatic β-cells culminate in β-cell apoptosis, which further reinforces the control of metabolism by insulin resistance. FAs are converted to acetyl-CoA through the process of beta-oxidation, in diabetic patients, and excessive and uncontrolled hepatic glucose synthesis elevates blood sugar levels [63].

This state indicates that the body is under the control of insulin-resistant hormones and uses FAs to provide energy to the liver in the absence of absolute or relative insulin [66]. FAs that are not β-oxidized by the liver is esterified by glycerol, coupled to apoB100 and transported into the blood. The reason for elevated plasma TGs in obese individuals with insulin-controlled reverse metabolism is that these large VLDL accumulate in the blood without their TGs being digested, and low levels of HDL cholesterol are another characteristic of obese people under insulin control [63, 67].

10. Conclusions

Obesity is defined as generalized increase in adipose tissue. It is a systemic illness which affects various body organs, resulting in metabolic deterioration, characterized by inflammatory processes, expressed according to the interactions between the genome and the environment, and manifest phenotypically as increased deposition of adipose tissue. Adipose tissue has the ability to buffer the surplus of energy through lipid storage through the expansion of this tissue, which is a sign of proper functionality.

Increased adipocytokines resulting from hyperplasia, proliferation, and differentiation of preadipocytes are responsible for controlling the physiological response of adipose tissue. When the subcutaneous adipose tissue does not adequately store the energy surplus due to exceeding storage capacity, the visceral fat depot expands with decrease in lipogenesis and increased adipocyte hypertrophy.

Acknowledgements

This work has been self-financed by the authors.

Conflict of interest

The authors declare no conflict of interest.

Author details

Maritza Torres Valdez[1*] and Valmore José Bermúdez Pirela[2]

1 Ministry of Public Health of Ecuador, Climedic, Cuenca, Ecuador

2 Universidad Simón Bolívar, Cúcuta, Colombia

*Address all correspondence to: torres.maritza78@yahoo.es

References

[1] Gutiérrez Cortez EA, Goicochea Ríos E del S, Linares Reyes E. Definition of obesity: Beyond the body mass index. Rev. MEDICA VALLEJIANA/Vallejian Med J. 2020;**9**:61-64

[2] Rolim LA, FCM DS, Chaves LL, Gonçalves MLCM, Freitas-Neto JL, Nascimento AL, et al. The colors of adipose tissue. Nature. 2020:539-547

[3] Rolim LA, FCM DS, Chaves LL, Gonçalves MLCM, Freitas-Neto JL, Nascimento AL, et al. Adipose tissue: Immune function and alterations caused by obesity. Nature. 2020:539-547

[4] Rodríguez A, Echandía C, Sánchez A, Satizábal JM, Montoya JC, García VF. Complexity of obesity-associated gene expression in human adipose tissue. Rev. Med. 2019:14-25

[5] Hernández Sandoval G, Rivera Valbuena J, Serrano Uribe R, Villalta Gómez D, Abbate León M, Acosta Núñez L, et al. Visceral adiposity, pathogenesis and measurement. Rev. Venez Endocrinol y Metab. 2017;**15**:70-77

[6] Izaola O, de Luis D, Sajoux I, Domingo JC, Vidal M. Inflammation and obesity (Lipoinflammation). Nutr Hosp. 2015;**31**:2352-2358

[7] Montalvo CE. Adipose Tissue. Department of Cell and Tissue Biology, School of Medicine, National Autonomous University of Mexico; 2010. pp. 1-7

[8] Ruiz-Ojeda FJ, Méndez-Gutiérrez A, Aguilera CM, Plaza-Díaz J. Extracellular matrix remodeling of adipose tissue in obesity and metabolic diseases. Int J Mol Sci. 2019;**20**:4888

[9] de Neto IV S, Durigan JLQ, da Silva ASR, de Marqueti RC. Adipose tissue extracellular matrix remodeling in response to dietary patterns and exercise: Molecular landscape, mechanistic insights, and therapeutic approaches. Biology (Basel). 2022;**11**:765

[10] Elias CP, Antunes DE, Coelho MS, De Lima CL, Rassi N, De Melo APM, et al. Evaluation of the hypothalamic–pituitary–adrenal axis in a case series of familial partial lipodystrophy 11 medical and health sciences 1103 clinical sciences. Diabetol Metab Syndr. BioMed Central. 2019;**11**:1-8. DOI: 10.1186/s13098-018-0396-4

[11] Davidson M, Priya PV. General Overview of Lipid Metabolism. MSD Man; 2021. pp. 1-4

[12] Suárez-Carmona W, Sánchez-Oliver AJ, González-Jurado JA. Pathophysiology of obesity: Current perspective. Rev. Chil Nutr. 2017;**44**:226-233

[13] Tozzi M, Novak I. Purinergic receptors in adipose tissue as potential targets in metabolic disorders. Front Pharmacol. 2017;**8**:1-8

[14] Bermudez V, Rojas J, Aguirre M, Cano C, Arraiz N, Silva C, et al. The sick adipocyte theory: The forces of clustering at glance. In: Role Adipocyte Dev Type 2 Diabetes. London, UK: IntechOpen; 2011

[15] Bermúdez V, Durán P, Rojas E, Díaz MP, Rivas J, Nava M, et al. The sick adipose tissue: New insights into defective signaling and crosstalk with the myocardium. Front Endocrinol (Lausanne). 2021;**12**:1-15

[16] Gómez-Romero P, Alarcón-Sotelo A, Rodríguez-Weber F, Díaz-Greene E.

Adiponectin as a therapeutic target. Med Interna Mex. 2017;**33**:770-777

[17] Inoue T, Uchida T, Kamishirado H, Sakuma M, Sakai Y, Takayanagi K, et al. Possible relationship between insulin resistance and remnant-like lipoprotein particles in coronary endothelial dysfunction. Clin Cardiol. Foundation for Advances in Medicine and Science Inc.;. 2002;**25**:532-536

[18] Rojas E, Rodríguez-molina D, Bolli P. The role of adiponectin in endothelial dysfunction and hypertension. Curr Hypertens Rep. 2014;**16**(8):463

[19] Achari AE, Jain SK. Adiponectin, a therapeutic target for obesity, diabetes, and endothelial dysfunction. Int J Mol Sci. 2017;**18**:1321

[20] J Ram, G Sp, H Pag, Mál, Solis-Sáinz Juan C. Brown adipose tissue proliferation and activation as a possible tool against obesity. 2021

[21] Kazak L, Chouchani ET, Stavrovskaya IG, Lu GZ, Jedrychowski MP, Egan DF, et al. UCP1 deficiency causes brown fat respiratory chain depletion and sensitizes mitochondria to calcium overload-induced dysfunction. Proc Natl Acad Sci U S A. 2017;**114**:7981-7986

[22] Ouchi N, Kihara S, Arita Y, Okamoto Y. Basic science reports endothelial NF- B signaling through a. Intern Med. 2000;**1296-301**

[23] Saito M, Matsushita M, Yoneshiro T, Okamatsu-Ogura Y. Brown adipose tissue, diet-induced thermogenesis, and Thermogenic food ingredients: From mice to men. Front Endocrinol (Lausanne). 2020;**11**:222

[24] Wu J, Cohen P, Spiegelman BM. Adaptive thermogenesis in adipocytes: Is beige the new brown? Genes Dev. 2013;**27**:234-250

[25] Salazar J, Luzardo E, Mejías JC, Rojas J, Ferreira A, Rivas-ríos JR, et al. Epicardial fat: Physiological. Pathological, and Therapeutic Implications. 2016;**2016**:14-16

[26] Talman AH, Psaltis PJ, Cameron JD, Meredith IT, Seneviratne SK, Wong DTL. Epicardial adipose tissue: Far more than a fat depot. Cardiovasc Diagn Ther. 2014;**4**:416-429

[27] Oliva Lorenzo L. Effect of the proportion of dietary components on different aspects of rat metabolism in a context of obesity. 2019. Available from: https://widgets.ebscohost.com/prod/customerspecific/ns000545/customproxy.php?url=https://search.ebscohost.com/login.aspx?direct=true&db=edstdx&AN=edstdx.10803.667435&amp%0Alang=pt-pt&site=eds-live&scope=site

[28] Iacobellis G. Epicardial adipose tissue in contemporary cardiology. Vol. 19. USA: Springer; 2022. pp. 593-606

[29] Romieu I, Dossus L, Barquera S, Blottière HM, Franks PW, Gunter M, et al. Energy balance and obesity: What are the main drivers? Cancer Causes Control. Springer International Publishing. 2017;**28**:247-258

[30] Spanish Society Of Biochemistry And Molecular Biology. Obesity Bochemistry. SEBBM [Internet]. 2016. Available from: http://www.ub.edu/tam/documents/Dossier Biochemistry of obesity des2016.pdf

[31] Longo M, Zatterale F, Naderi J, Parrillo L, Formisano P, Raciti GA, et al. Adipose tissue dysfunction as determinant of obesity-associated metabolic complications. Int J Mol Sci. 2019;**20**:2358

[32] González Maglio DH, Paz ML, Leoni J. Sunlight effects on immune system: Is there something Else in addition to UV-induced immunosuppression? Biomed Res Int. 2016;**2016**:1934518

[33] Hall KD, Farooqi IS, Friedman JM, Klein S, Loos RJF, Mangelsdorf DJ, et al. The energy balance model of obesity: Beyond calories in, calories out. Am J Clin Nutr. 2022;**115**:1243-1254

[34] Sohn JW. Network of hypothalamic neurons that control appetite. BMB Rep. 2015;**48**:229-233

[35] Forouzanfar MH, Afshin A, Alexander LT, Anderson HR, Bhutta ZA, Biryukov S, et al. Global, regional, and national comparative risk assessment of 79 behavioural, environmental and occupational, and metabolic risks or clusters of risks, 1990-2015: A systematic analysis for the global burden of disease study 2015. Lancet. 2016;**388**:1659-1724

[36] Ross FA, MacKintosh C, Hardie DG. AMP-activated protein kinase: A cellular energy sensor that comes in 12 flavours. FEBS J. 2016;**283**:2987-3001

[37] López M. Hypothalamic AMPK and energy balance. Eur J Clin Invest. 2018;**48**:e12996

[38] Zatterale F, Longo M, Naderi J, Raciti GA, Desiderio A, Miele C, et al. Chronic adipose tissue inflammation linking obesity to insulin resistance and type 2 diabetes. Front Physiol. 2020;**10**:1-20

[39] Mechanick JI, Hurley DL, Garvey WT. Adiposity-based chronic disease as a new diagnostic term: The American association of clinical endocrinologists and American college of endocrinology position statement. Endocr Pract. 2017;**23**:372-378

[40] Liu R, Nikolajczyk BS. Tissue immune cells fuel obesity-associated inflammation in adipose tissue and beyond. Front Immunol. 2019;**10**:1587

[41] Patel P, Abate N. Role of subcutaneous adipose tissue in the pathogenesis of insulin resistance. J Obes. 2013;**2013**:489187

[42] Manna P, Jain SK. Obesity, oxidative stress, adipose tissue dysfunction, and the associated health risks: Causes and therapeutic strategies. Metab Syndr Relat Disord. 2015;**13**:423-444

[43] Thomas D, Caroline M, Apovian M. Macrophage functions in lean and obese adipose tissue. HHS Public Acces. 2017;**72**:120-143

[44] Caslin HL, Bhanot M, Bolus WR, Hasty A, Francisco S. Bioenergetics in Obesity. 2021;**295**:101-113

[45] Surmi BK, Hasty AH. Macrophage infiltration into adipose tissue. Future Lipidol [Internet]. 2008;**3**:545-556

[46] Sproston NR, Ashworth JJ. Role of C-reactive protein at sites of inflammation and infection. Front Immunol. 2018;**9**:1-11

[47] Rojas J, Salazar J, Martínez MS, Palmar J, Bautista J, Chávez-Castillo M, et al. Macrophage heterogeneity and plasticity: Impact of macrophage biomarkers on atherosclerosis. Scientifica (Cairo). 2015;**2015**:1-17

[48] Lin P, Ji HH, Li YJ, Guo SD. Macrophage plasticity and atherosclerosis therapy. Front Mol Biosci. 2021;**8**:1-21

[49] Ma B, Yang Y, Li Z, Zhao D, Zhang W, Jiang Y, et al. Modular bioinformatics analysis demonstrates that a toll-like receptor signaling pathway is involved in the regulation of

macrophage polarization. Mol Med Rep. 2018;**18**:4313-4320

[50] Li C, Levin M, Kaplan DL. Bioelectric modulation of macrophage polarization. Sci Rep. 2016;**6**:1-12. DOI: 10.1038/srep21044

[51] Pérez-Pérez A, Sánchez-Jiménez F, Vilariño-García T, Sánchez-Margalet V. Role of leptin in inflammation and vice versa. Int J Mol Sci. 2020;**21**:1-24

[52] Chait A, den Hartigh LJ. Adipose tissue distribution, inflammation and its metabolic consequences, including diabetes and cardiovascular disease. Front Cardiovasc Med. 2020;**7**:1-41

[53] Boucher J, Kleinridders A, Kahn CR. Insulin receptor signaling in Normal. Cold Spring Harb Perspect Biol. 2014;**2014**(6):a009191

[54] Liu H, Du T, Li C, Yang G. STAT3 phosphorylation in central leptin resistance. Nutr Metab [Internet]. BioMed Central. 2021;**18**:1-13. DOI: 10.1186/s12986-021-00569-w

[55] Wunderlich CM, Hövelmeyer N, Wunderlich FT. Mechanisms of chronic JAK-STAT3-SOCS3 signaling in obesity. JAKSTAT. 2013;**2**:e23878

[56] Tejero J, Shiva S, Gladwin MT. Sources of vascular nitric oxide and reactive oxygen species and their regulation. Physiol Rev. 2019;**99**:311-379

[57] Han J, Kaufman RJ. The role of ER stress in lipid metabolism and lipotoxicity. J Lipid Res. 2016, ASBMB. Currently published by Elsevier Inc.; originally published by American Society for Biochemistry and Molecular Biology. **57**:1329-1338. DOI: 10.1194/jlr.R067595

[58] Röder PV, Wu B, Liu Y, Han W. Pancreatic regulation of glucose homeostasis. Exp Mol Med. 2016;**48**:e219

[59] Tronoso PC, Amaya JP. Social factors In the eating behaviors of university university students. 2009

[60] Moreno Salazar SF. Selected Topics in General Biochemistry. Topics Sel Biochemistry Gen [Internet]. 2019. 132. Available from: http://www.dagus.uson.mx/smoreno/8 Metabolism.pdf

[61] Cano R, Villalobos M, Aguirre M, Corzo G, Ferreira A. From obesity to diabetes: Insulin-resistance is a defense mechanism and not a disease. 2017;**1**:20-28

[62] Ježek P, Jabůrek M, Holendová B, Plecitá-Hlavatá L. Fatty acid-stimulated insulin secretion vs. lipotoxicity. Molecules. 2018;**23**:1483

[63] Pant R, Firmal P, Shah VK, Alam A, Chattopadhyay S. Epigenetic regulation of Adipogenesis in development of metabolic syndrome. Front Cell Dev Biol. 2021;**8**:619888

[64] Kasselman LJ, Vernice NA, DeLeon J, Reiss AB. The gut microbiome and elevated cardiovascular risk in obesity and autoimmunity. Atherosclerosis. 2018;**271**:203-213

[65] Hatting M, Tavares CDJ, Sharabi K, Rines AK, Puigserver P. Insulin regulation of gluconeogenesis. Ann N Y Acad Sci. 2018;**1411**:21-35

[66] Alves-Bezerra M, Cohen DE. Triglyceride metabolism in the liver. Compr Physiol. 2018;**8**:1-22

[67] Amaral G, Bushee J, Cordani UG, Kawashita K, Reynolds JH, Ffmde A, et al. National Health and Nutrition Survey ENSANUT. Instituto Nacional de Salud Pública; 2012. pp. 180-186

Chapter 4

Diet-Induced Overweight Conditions: Effect on Brain Structure, Cognitive Function, and Neurogenesis

Amina Khatun, Surendra Patra, Kuntal Ghosh, Shrabani Pradhan and Sudipta Chakrabarti

Abstract

Obesity, a chronic condition that is currently prevalent in both developed and developing nations, is associated with pathological features that ultimately put individuals at risk for a number of negative health issues. Cognitive decline and insulin resistance are two aspects of metabolic syndrome that are closely linked to neurological dysfunction during obesity. Several studies suggest that obesity is associated with regional structural changes, especially signs of cortical thinning in specific brain regions like the hippocampus, and reduced microstructural integrity of the white matter tract is associated with an overall lower academic performance. Obesity causes a loss of brain size and volume indicating a loss of neurons which leads to poor cognitive performance and reduced neurogenesis. An increase in the production of free fatty acids seen with HFD eating might result in increased oxidative stress and increased production of reactive oxygen species. The main cause of systemic inflammation in obesity is the build-up of adipose as it releases TNFα, PAI-1, CRP, IL-1β, and IL-6 which contribute to a pro-inflammatory state in the central nervous system. These elements can all lead to the central IKK/NF-B inflammatory signalling cascade being activated, which can cause a vicious inflammatory cycle that quickens and causes neurodegeneration and cognitive decline.

Keywords: obesity, oxidative stress, inflammation, neurodegeneration, cognitive loss

1. Introduction

Overweight/obesity, a disease condition currently reaching epidemic proportions, particularly in industrialised countries, and linked to pathological changes that ultimately put people at risk for a variety of adverse health effects [1]. Obesity results from the accumulation of excessive body fat due to the consumption of excessive calories and is typically fuelled by western food habits and a sedentary lifestyle [2]. Food that has been processed and refined typically contains saturated fats, added sugar, and salts, which over long-term contribute to increased calorie intake. There is much speculation and considerable debate about whether obesity-associated cognitive function is a result of weight gain, or whether it is a result of behaviours that lead to weight gain (such as hedonic overeating) [3, 4]. Body mass index (BMI) 25 and 30 are the World Health Organisation's (WHO) definitions of overweight and obesity, respectively [5]. Body mass index (BMI, kg/m^2), which divides weight (kg) by height squared (m^2), is widely used to determine obesity. Based on BMI, there are three categories: normal weight (BMI 18.5–24.9 kg/m^2), overweight (BMI 25.0–29.9 kg/m^2), and obese (BMI 30.0 kg/m^2).

However, metabolic syndromes arise when caloric intake significantly outweighs expenditure while there is a sustained lack of physical activity. The presence of low-grade metabolic inflammation in visceral adipose tissue is also considered to be a primary component of metabolic syndrome, which is characterised by central obesity [6]. The metabolic syndrome consists of a number of risk factors that contribute to chronic non-communicable disorders such as cardiovascular diseases (CVD), type 2 diabetes, dyslipidaemia and hypertension as well as other diseases. In addition to CVD, obesity has also been linked to pathological changes in brain morphology and function and cognitive impairments [7]. Even though the central nervous system (CNS) and the peripheral nervous system (PNS) have very different structures and functions, both are vulnerable to the deleterious effects of obesity, indicating that visceral adiposity may facilitate a common pathophysiologic mechanism. The metabolic syndrome includes components that are strongly associated with neurological dysfunction, such as insulin resistance and hypertension leading to cognitive decline. Such factors are generated by obesity. As a result, several processes may be working together to cause neurological dysfunction, while it can be difficult to determine the precise impact of visceral adiposity on neurological dysfunction. Animal obesity models' mechanistic insights reveal that excessive dietary fat impairs the hypothalamic coordination of energy homeostasis [8]. This pathway may be associated with the disintegration of adipose tissue, resulting in increased levels of free fatty acids, systemic inflammation and dyslipidaemia. As a consequence of chronic calorie overconsumption, circulating triglycerides increase and are adversely affected by numerous organs, including the liver. Dyslipidaemia caused by free fatty acids can result in neurological dysfunction because of lipotoxicity and altered intracellular signalling. Despite these mechanisms affecting the CNS and PNS in multiple ways, obesity is known to have neurological complications [9].

While wide range of functions in human brain requires significant energy, there are limited energy stores in the brain, and those stores can meet only a portion of its energy requirements. The blood-brain barrier (BBB) allows nutrients to continuously enter the brain from the blood, which is how the brain obtains the necessary energy for optimal functioning. Under physiological circumstances, the brain's primary fuel source is glucose [10]. During development, and at times when glucose supply is insufficient, the brain can use alternative energy substrates such as ketone bodies, triglycerides, as well as lactate [11]. Several recent studies have demonstrated that nutrition and dietary intake have a profound effect on cognition, neuronal function, neuronal signalling, and synaptic plasticity [12, 13]. The consumption of diets rich in saturated fats has consistently been linked to impaired cognitive function, both in clinical and preclinical studies [14, 15]. It is of interest to note that adult studies suggest that consuming high-fat diets (HFD) on a short-term basis may impair attention and memory capabilities [16, 17]. Remarkably, consumption of a diet high in saturated fats is frequently cited as a cause of the cognitive decline and the development of Alzheimer's Disease [18]. Conversely, it has been suggested that diets high in polyunsaturated fatty acids enhance cognitive health Disease [18–20]. Depending on the composition, abundance, or lack of particular nutrients, the brain can be affected in different ways by different nutrient requirements. There is a known association between consuming saturated fat-rich diets and metabolic and cardiovascular diseases [21–23]. According to a growing body of research, obese individuals, and those with diabetes and with hypertension are at high risk of developing cognitive impairments and Alzheimer's disease [18, 24–27]. Since the global burden of both neurological diseases and metabolic disorders is increasing, it is necessary to investigate common underlying mechanisms associated with these rapidly increasing disease entities. In this article, we discuss how diet-induced overweight/obesity affect the function, neurogenesis and brain composure.

2. Overweight/obesity: the pathophysiology

In addition to storing energy and releasing it, adipose tissue serves as an insulation system for internal organs and a protection against trauma. Adipokines mediate the endocrine function of adipose tissue through hormones, cytokines, acute phase reactants, and growth factors [28]. These molecules play an important role in maintaining energy homeostasis along with the liver, pancreas, and brain. The major mechanism for achieving energy balance is via controlling energy intake and energy expenditure. Calories are truly calories, and they are all equal according to this fundamental energetic equation [29]. However, when we consider the pathophysiology of obesity-related comorbidities in addition to this merely energy balance aspect, we see that not all calories are created equal [29]. In order to properly explain the pathophysiology of obesity, two simultaneous discussions—one from an energy perspective and the other from a nutritional perspective—must be included. Here, we primarily concentrate on the second because there is controversy regarding the optimal nutritional composition, whereas there is significant agreement on the principles of energy balance management [6, 30]. Managing obesity-related diseases, such as CVD, requires a clear understanding of obesity-independent and obesity-dependent pathophysiologic effects.

Based on genome-wide association studies (GWAS), more than 140 chromosomal regions are associated with obesity [31]. The central nervous system has a significantly enriched gene expression profile associated with BMI and overall obesity [32]. Nevertheless, only a small number of genes, have been found to have a significant impact on BMI thus far. These are the paternally expressed genes along a specific region of chromosome 15 that cause Prader-Willi syndrome, as well as the genes that encode elements of leptin and melanocortin signalling [33]. Most researchers concur that environment, lifestyle, and genetic predisposition contribute to obesity predisposition [34]. Scientists generally agree that increased body weight or adiposity is actively regulated and mitigated by the body under constant environmental conditions, regardless of short-term perturbations in weight or adiposity [35]. Researchers have found that obesity is often defended as a disease, diverting blame from the person to the body's physiology, just as it is for normal-weight subjects [36]. In addition to adipocytes, adipose tissue contains stromovascular compartments, which are made up of nerve endings, blood vessels, preadipocytes, fibroblasts, endothelial cells, and resident immune cells [37]. As fat-storing cells, adipocytes store triglyceride-rich lipid droplets as a source of energy. Insulin is primarily responsible for regulating adipocyte energy uptake and storage, as it mediates fatty acid influx and lipogenesis while

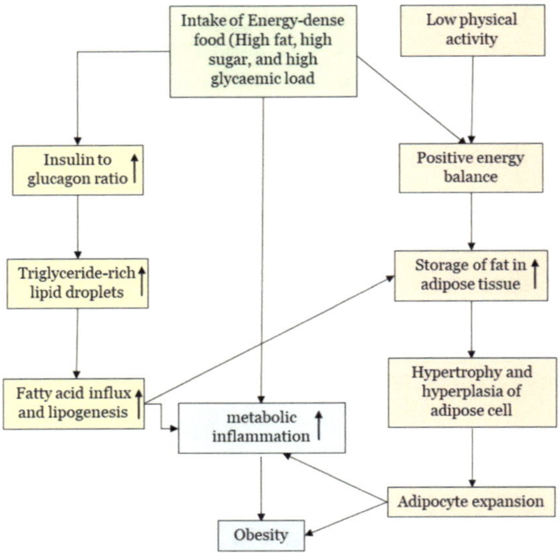

Figure 1.
Pathophysiology of obesity.

inhibiting lipolysis [38]. When adipocytes are in a negative energy balance, sympathetic neural stimulation promotes lipolysis of stored triglycerides where fatty acids are delivered into the bloodstream to feed non-adipose tissues [39]. The adipocyte undergoes hypertrophy (enlargement of adipocytes) or hyperplasia (proliferation and differentiation) when there is a positive energy balance (i.e., excess caloric intake), it causes the adipocytes to expand in order to store excess calories.

Low-grade metabolic inflammation is associated with increased adipose mass, especially visceral depots, which promote metabolic disease as a consequence of malfunctioning adipose tissue. By increasing adipose mass, especially in visceral depots, metabolic inflammation is linked to metabolic disease, which occurs when adipose tissues malfunction [6]. Adipose tissue inflammation has negative effects on adipokine release, insulin signalling, triglyceride accumulation, and basal lipolysis, among other things. These alterations produce peripheral-tissue and nervous system dysfunction because they result in elevated levels of circulating adipokines and free fatty acids Smith [40]. A chronic caloric surplus that triggers stress signalling pathways and activates local macrophages causes metabolic inflammation, which mostly affects hypertrophied adipose tissue resulting overweight and obesity (**Figure 1**).

3. The relationship between obesity and structural and functional changes in the brain

Various structural changes in the brain can be measured by changes in brain volume or density. Several studies suggest that obesity is associated with regional structural changes, especially in elderly populations [41]. Researchers have reported reduced frontal lobe, anterior cingulate gyrus, hippocampus, and thalamus volume in cognitively healthy obese older individuals. Middle-aged adults and the elderly with high BMI have also been found to have impaired frontal lobe integrity [42–44]. The volume and density of the brain are often used as indicators of structural changes.

A growing body of evidence indicates obesity is associated with regional structural changes in obese populations, especially in elderly people [41]. The hippocampus, cingulate gyrus, and frontal lobes of obese older individuals were found to have reduced volume according to a tensor-based morphometry study [44]. Middle-aged adults and the elderly with high BMI have also been shown to have damage to their frontal lobes [42, 43]. The presence of obesity has been also linked to global structural changes in the brain, including an overall reduction in grey matter and white matter volumes [44].

Grey matter volume structural anomalies in obese patients were discovered by a recent systematic review [45]. The left middle frontal gyrus left middle temporal gyrus, left amygdala, and left cerebellar hemisphere all showed a consistent decline in grey matter in obese people when compared to the control regions, according to an analysis of 10 research published up to December 2017 [41, 43, 46–53]. A study by Kurth et al. found that the superior frontal gyrus on the left, middle and inferior frontal gyri, the right frontal pole, the left insula, as well as the bilateral superior and middle temporal gyri were negatively affected by body mass index [54]. According to García García et al., obesity and body mass are associated with significantly less grey matter volume in the areas of the brain that play a crucial role in executive control [55]. Obesity-related factors are consistently linked to decreased grey matter volume in a number of regions, including the left temporal pole, bilateral cerebellum, and medial prefrontal cortex. Similar to lean and overweight persons with increasing BMI, obese people have less total grey matter volume. Yokum et al., found that future weight increase is associated with a reduced amount of grey matter in the areas involved in inhibitory regulation [56]. Weight gain is primarily the result of abnormalities in the white matter volumes of the regional spine, not in the grey matter volumes, whereas abnormalities in grey matter volumes increase the likelihood of weight gain in the future.

Similarly, here is compelling evidence that people with increased BMI experience a brain-wide white matter decrease [57, 58]. The result is in line with a major investigation that found links between increased BMI and decreased white matter integrity in two separate, sizable populations [59]. Uncinate fascicle, internal capsule, corticospinal tract, inferior fronto-occipital fascicle, inferior and superior longitudinal fascicles, corpus callosum (cingulate gyrus and hippocampus), and cingulum are just a few of the white matter regions that are known to decrease with a higher BMI [45, 48, 50]. The critical limbic structures are connected to the prefrontal regions by local changes in the white matter fibre tracts linked to greater BMI, which may help to explain why obesity in older age is associated with an increased risk for cognitive impairments and dementia [60]. Obese people could age more quickly than average people, which is thought to raise the risk of cognitive impairment [61]. The fibre tracts that link limbic systems to prefrontal regions are the most commonly affected. These abnormalities are indicative of a loss of white matter integrity brought on by demyelination or inflammatory effects, and can be described by axonal injury or cellular death [61]. The bilateral thalamus, putamen, and globus pallidus in obese individuals are larger than those of normal weight, although the bilateral caudate is smaller [62]. Even obese people (with a BMI of 25 to 30 kg/m^2) have symptoms of basal ganglia atrophy and radiating crown [44].

Yau et al. [63] found evidence of cortical thinning in some areas of the brain and decreased microstructural quality of the white matter circuit in obese adolescents. In this study, obese youths performed no worse in cognitive tests than non-obese youths, but structural impairments were associated with a lower academic performance overall [63]. While these findings, do not prove causality, it is biologically conceivable to connect brain anatomical alterations to impaired cognitive function. Poor cognitive performance can be linked causally to smaller brain sizes and volumes since these changes are suggestive of a loss of neurons. Adolescents who are obese may show signs of brain abnormalities, but it may take them until later in life for these changes to cause cognitive impairment. In the early phases of cognitive decline, advanced brain imaging techniques that are more likely to detect anatomical micro alterations do not immediately translate into cognitive dysfunction [64]. As a result, it is particularly important to examine how obesity affects brain function by integrating physiological assessment with cognitive tests. Van Opstal [65] investigated the impact of weight loss (sustained fasting) on brain function in obese persons [65]. Fourteen subjects in this study met the BMI criteria for being classified as obese. During an overnight fast, a 48-hour fast, and an 8-week weight loss programme, brain imaging data were collected using whole-brain resting-state functional magnetic resonance imaging (MRI). The weight loss intervention, according to the researchers, decreased activation in the brain regions in charge of salience, sensory-motor control, and executive control, indicating a connection between weight loss and changes in neurological activity brought on by obesity [65].

A recent meta-analysis on anomalies in brain structure and obesity was undertaken by Opel et al. who also took into account the effects of ageing, hereditary risk, and psychiatric problems [66]. This study involved 6420 participants and examined the relationship between obesity (BMI > 30 kg/m^2) and brain anatomy. Results showed a strong relationship between obesity and cortical and subcortical abnormalities, particularly in the lower temporal-frontal cortex thickness. Cortical thickness was influenced by the combination of age and a higher polygenic risk score [66].

4. Cognitive effects of diet-induced obesity/overweight

Cognitive impairment can be caused by obesity when the physiology of the human energy system is impaired. In addition to affecting cognition and the Central Nervous System (CNS), obesity may also affect verbal learning, executive function, and decision-making [67]. An individual's cognitive function plays an important role in acquiring knowledge and information through the constant use of language, memory, and attention [68]. The effects of obesity on cognitive function can be attributed to structural and functional changes in the brain [69–71]. In executive functioning tests, obese females performed worse than normal-weight females. There was a reduction in grey matter volume in the left orbitofrontal region associated with a decrease in executive functioning [71]. Older people who are obese during midlife are more likely to develop dementia [72]. Several CVD risks factors, including obesity, T2D, dyslipidaemia, and hypertension, were demonstrated to negatively impact cognition in a systematic review [73]. According to studies, older women who have more body fat have poorer cognitive functioning [71].

5. Childhood obesity and cognitive functions

With childhood obesity is currently on the rise, deficits in attention and cognitive flexibility have been linked to childhood obesity [74]. According to cross-sectional research on overweight children, overweight status was linked to worse test scores, particularly in the areas of arithmetic, reading, and executive function, while being physically fit was linked to better cognition performance, and behaviour [75]. Children who are overweight struggle with spatial cognitive tasks, and studies have revealed variations in both motor and mental rotation efficiency [76]. When rotation activities were challenging, overweight children made more mistakes than children of average weight [76]. Obesity can affect cognitive abilities, particularly executive abilities, in children and adolescents [77, 78]. According to studies, adolescents who are obese have lower executive and attentional cognitive abilities [79, 80]. Insufficient cognitive domains, including executive function and attention deficits, were found in obese adolescents in pilot research [79].

Data analysis from the general population revealed links between gender-specific features of developmental functioning with obesity and impairment [81]. Infants with high subcutaneous fat and children who are overweight or obese had delayed motor development [82]. It has been demonstrated that overweight children have significantly worse perceived and actual physical competence [83]. Overweight children had varying levels of difficulty with basic motor skills [84]. Compared to their peers who were of a healthy weight, obese children reported reduced degrees of gross motor function. The most significant variations were found in balance and locomotor abilities [85]. In comparison to children who were of a healthy weight, children who were overweight performed less effectively in the domains of intelligence, coordination, and gross motor abilities [86]. Significant abnormalities in gross and fine motor skills related to weight were observed in obese children [87].

5.1 Possible mechanisms for cognitive impairment driven by diet-induced overweight

5.1.1 Role of oxidative stress on cognitive impairment

The brain is thought to be the organ most susceptible to harm from oxidative stress [88]. This is explained by the greater lipid content, the high oxygen demand, and the scarcity of antioxidant enzymes [11]. Consistent overnutrition brought on by HFD diet may result in an abundance of reactive oxygen species (ROS) and reactive nitrogen species (RNS) [89]. Because of the excessive production of these species, macromolecules like DNA, membrane lipids, and protein structures are harmed [90]. Reduced glutathione, catalase, and superoxide dismutase act as endogenous antioxidant enzymes to neutralise these free radicals. A high fat diet causes excessive ROS production that exceeds the antioxidant enzymes' capacity [91].

Here, it is briefly mentioned how an HFD diet might leads to increased oxidative stress. HFD consumption results in an increase in free fatty acid production. In the normal diet-feeding process, electrons are transferred from cofactors (NADH and FADH2) to complex I of the mitochondrial respiratory chain, where they combine safely with oxygen and protons to form water [92]. Free fatty acids are then oxidised in the mitochondria through the mitochondrial respiratory chain. Superoxide radicals are created when some of these electrons interact with oxygen. Conversely, HFD feeding results in increased mitochondrial -oxidation of FFAs, resulting in increased levels of superoxide anion and an excess electron flow [92, 93]. The natural antioxidant enzymes can also be consumed by ROS, which increases the risk of oxidative injury to the brain [92, 94]. According to a growing body of research, the development of cognitive decline and increased oxidative stress may be correlated, [95–98]. These findings suggest that increased oxidative stress is a major contributor to the cognitive abnormalities caused by HFD.

Many studies have demonstrated that HFD eating causes the levels of oxidative stress indicators in the brain to increase [99–104]. One of the most delicate areas of the brain to suffer from selective oxidative stress damage is the neocortex and hippocampal region. The impairment of cognition is also closely related to hippocampal oxidative stress [105–108]. Researchers have used antioxidant therapy to demonstrate cognitive benefits in support of the idea that oxidative stress may be a potential mechanism underlying the cognitive impairment associated with HFD eating. In HFD-fed mice, deficiencies can be restored by employing this strategy [99, 109, 110].

5.1.2 Role of neuroinflammation on cognitive impairment

Inflammation is controlled in a variety of ways by macrophages, depending on their differentiation level. Traditionally activated macrophages (M1) release proinflammatory cytokines and reactive oxygen species (ROS) to initiate an immune response, whereas alternatively activated macrophages (M2) reduce inflammation, promote tissue remodelling, and release growth factors in the later stages of an immune response [111]. Adipose tissue macrophages in healthy, nonobese humans appear to act similarly to M2 macrophages in that they contain arginase, which limits nitric oxide synthesis and promotes polyamine synthesis, and they release little to no proinflammatory cytokines [112]. Chemokine CCL2, formerly called monocyte chemotactic protein-1 (MCP1), is released by macrophages. TNF and IL-6 are also macrophage-released cytokines [113]. It is possible for M1 and M2 macrophages to coexist, which might result in fibrosis and prolonged inflammation [114]. Systemic inflammation in obesity is the result of build-up of adipose tissue and the increase in the levels of tumour necrosis factor-alpha (TNF-α), plasminogen activator inhibitor-1, C-reactive protein, interleukin-1-beta (IL-1β), and interleukin-6 (IL-6), Adipose tissue, particularly lymphocytes and macrophages, contains hypertrophic adipocytes and immune cells that contribute to inflammation [115, 116]. It is possible that processes of necrotic clearance are similar to inflammatory responses mediated by M1 in obese individuals [117, 118]. Macrophages release chemokines like CC-chemokine ligand 2 (CCL2; formerly known as monocyte chemotactic protein-1 (MCP1)) and cytokines like TNF and IL-6. Type 2 diabetes (T2DM) might result from interference in insulin signalling pathway in adipocytes caused by TNF and IL-6 [119]. Over time, macrophages build up in adipose tissue, and the cytokines they release can cause insulin resistance and T2DM [112, 113]. These inflammatory macrophages can increase atherogenic and CVD risks that are a feature of the metabolic syndrome associated with obesity by overexpressing procoagulant proteins [119].

5.1.3 Effects of gut dysbiosis on obesity-related disorders

Abnormalities in neurochemistry and inflammation may also be caused by the gut microbiota associated with obesity [120, 121]. The modification of the gut microbiota, or dysbiosis, can help to explain obesity since it is a factor that is central to host physiology and environmental stressors (such as diet and lifestyle) [120].

Gut dysbiosis (imbalance in gut microbiota composition caused by host genetics, lifestyle, and exposure to microorganisms) may facilitate diet-induced obesity and metabolic complications through a variety of mechanisms, including immune dysregulation, altered energy regulation, altered gut hormone regulation, and proinflammatory mechanisms (such as lipopolysaccharide endotoxins that cross the gut barrier and enter the portal circulation) [121–123]. Recent studies have indicated that changes in the composition of the gut and inflammation brought on by a leaky gut may have an impact on the pathophysiology of many disorders, such as depression, chronic fatigue syndrome, obesity, and type 2 diabetes (T2DM) (a loss of intestinal barrier integrity that reduces the ability of the gut to protect the internal environment) [124].

Obesity-related inflammation can impact the amygdala, cerebral cortex, hippocampus, and brain stem [125]. Numerous routes, including alteration of the blood–brain barrier (BBB) and choroid plexuses, have been used to link obesity-related low-grade inflammation to neuroinflammation [126]. Insulin resistance is caused by peripheral inflammation, which is seen in obesity [112, 113]. Although it is widely acknowledged that the brain plays a special role in immunity, there have been some instances of transitions between peripheral and central inflammation. It is also possible to express adipokines in the CNS, where these factors have receptors. Adipose tissue produces adipokines, which are expressed in the CNS as well. Peripherally produced adipokines can influence the CNS by crossing the BBB or changing its physiology by interacting with the cells that make up the BBB [127]. There is a strong correlation between neuroinflammation and oxidative stress and a wide range of chronic neurodegenerative diseases [128]. These processes can be regulated by adipokines. Inflammation in the brain can also result from damage to the BBB with ageing [129]. The most significant contributor to cognitive dysfunction may be neuroinflammation, which might also act as a primary pathogenic mechanism for ageing [130].

There is a connection between the activation states of cytokines and chemokines produced by different cell types in adipose tissue outside the central nervous system (quiescent or activated). Obesity and neurodegeneration are linked via the production of inflammatory cytokines and resistance to insulin-like growth factor 1 (IGF-1) [115, 116, 128, 130, 131]. As a result of central inflammation in obesity, hypothalamic satiety signals are interrupted, which perpetuates overeating and has negative consequences for cognition [132]. Different disorders associated with ageing are also thought to be influenced by chronic inflammation. Peripheral inflammation and associated metabolic abnormalities promote T2DM, insulin resistance, and neurodegenerative diseases [133]. In the abdominal adipose tissue, macrophages promote the synthesis of cytokines and proinflammatory chemokines that can cross the BBB. Interferon-gamma can activate microglia, which then serve as relays for neuroinflammation [134].

A number of pathological mechanisms are exacerbated by hypertension, diabetes, and obesity, including cerebral hypoperfusion and glucose hypometabolism. Neuroinflammation and oxidative-nitrosative stress are triggered by these risk factors. There are several cycles of pathological feedback caused by proinflammatory cytokines, endothelin1, and oxidative-nitrosative stress [135]. These cascades cause neurodegeneration and an increase in neuronal $Ca2+$ [60]. Long-term damage to mitochondria, proteins, DNA, and fatty acids is promoted by oxidative-nitrosative stress. These elements magnify and sustain a variety of problematic feedback loops [136]. Chronic cerebral hypoperfusion results from dysfunctional energy metabolism (compromised mitochondrial ATP production), formation of -amyloid, endothelial dysfunction, and modification of the BBB [115, 130]. Hypoperfusion deprives the brain of oxygen and nutrition, which are its two most critical trophic factors. As a result, the brain experiences synaptic dysfunction and neuronal death, which causes grey and white matter atrophy [136]. The decline of M2 macrophages in the CNS is associated with many neurodegenerative diseases and the subsequent increase of M1-induced inflammation [134]. Microglia and macrophages express the macrophage-stimulating protein receptor (MST1R). In the periphery, obesity-mediated inflammation is attenuated by activating MST1R with its ligand, a macrophage-stimulating protein. Cleavage to the MST1R ligand in vivo regulates the activation of macrophage-dependent repair (M2) [137]. Apoptosis can be caused by neuroinflammation [138]. Its fundamental physiological function, which helps to maintain homeostasis, is a tightly controlled process of cell death. A variety of proteins, signal transducers, and signalling pathway cascades collaborate to fully implement apoptosis [139]. Numerous disorders' origin and/or progression are strongly correlated with poor apoptotic regulation [138, 140]. TRAIL, TNF, and Fas ligand (Fas-L) bind to the extracellular domain of DR (transmembrane receptors) to initiate the TNF pathway, the main apoptosis pathway [138–140]. During an inflammatory response, TNF- and Fas-L can cause certain neurons to apoptose [138].

Caspases, which are cysteine proteases, are activated during apoptosis, which controls all of the morphological changes that distinguish this type of cell death [138]. Activating effector caspases (caspases 3, 6, and 7) via a controlled, irreversible, and self-amplifying proteolytic route begins with activating initiator caspases (caspases 2, 8, or 10) [141].

6. Obesity and impaired neurogenesis

It has now been proven beyond a shadow of a doubt that neurogenesis takes place in specific parts of the adult brain, debunking the long-held belief that brain cells lack any capacity for regeneration [142]. Neuronal stem cells (NSCs) in the CNS of adult mammals may now be isolated and identified toas a result of advances in science and technology. Even though adult neurogenesis was first observed in the 1960s, multiple articles have argued that adult mammalian brains do not show any indications of neurogenesis [143–145]. Adult hippocampal neurogenesis in mammals, including rodents was not "rediscover[ed]" for another three decades [146, 147]. When these freshly produced cells' "stem-like" properties were first identified in the 1990s, it was believed that NSCs could auto replicate and give rise to a variety of neural lineages in adult mammalian brains, including neurons, astrocytes, and oligodendrocytes [148–150]. Later research showed that NSCs were mostly found in the subventricular zone (SVZ) of the lateral ventricles and the subgranular zone (SGZ) of the hippocampus dentate gyrus in the adult central CNS [151]. The functional integrity and plasticity of these brain regions are thought to be maintained by these adult NSCs by initiating neurogenesis in response to intrinsic and extrinsic changes, which is consistent with the observation that neurogenesis was also highly prevalent around these regions in adult mammalian brain [152]. Recent research indicates that multipotent NSCs, which have the capacity to differentiate into new neurons as well as astrocytes and oligodendrocytes, can be reprogrammed to grow in the adult mouse hypothalamus in the medio basal region of the hypothalamus (MBH) and the third ventricle wall [153]. These newly formed neurons in the adult mouse hypothalamus could integrate into the existing neuronal network and have recently been shown to be functionally active [154].

Several decades ago, neurogenesis in the adult brain was considered impossible and was refuted, but it has now been widely acknowledged as a very common phenomenon [146, 148]. Many brain regions are abundant in new neurons and NSCs [146].

DOI: http://dx.doi.org/10.5772/intechopen.110610

The hypothalamus, which houses the body's neuroendocrine system, has recently been found to be both a rich NSC niche and a hotspot of neurogenesis [153]. It is believed that these hypothalamic NSCs play a key role in the neuroendocrine modulation of whole-body physiology [155–157] as well as systemic ageing [158]. Through local or extrinsic insults to this hypothalamic region, disruption of their neurogenic function may lead to neurodegenerative manifestations across the neuronal milieu. A specific condition known as neurodegeneration, the loss of cognitive abilities, and hypothalamic stem cell damage, as well as obesity and chronic energy imbalance, have been reported to occur after chronic inflammation or inflammation induced by overnutrition or ageing. Additionally, there is data linking brain diseases to overnutrition. Neuroinflammation is clearly to blame for poor neurogenesis and NSC depletion [159]. Furthermore, chronic inflammation slows neurogenesis, NSC survival, and differentiation, and increases ageing-related decline and neurodegenerative disorders [158, 160–163] despite providing a necessary defensive mechanism for the body. IKB kinase (IKK) and its downstream nuclear transcription factor NFκB (IKK/NFκB signalling) are part of the proinflammatory axis in the hypothalamus that is exacerbated by overnutrition [60, 164]. It has been found that overeating and age-related activation of the IKK/NFκB signalling pathway all contribute to obesity, chronic energy imbalance, neurotoxicity and cognitive impairment 21, and hypothalamic stem cell degradation [164–169]. A connection between overnutrition/ageing-induced neuroinflammation and neurodegenerative diseases is further supported by evidence and implications relating to overnutrition-induced neurological diseases including Alzheimer's (AD) and Parkinson's (PD) [170–173].

While neuroinflammation is an important defence mechanism in reaction to infections, illnesses, and brain damage, persistent inflammation compromises the body's normal defences and promotes the progressive neurological and neurodegenerative illnesses [160–163]. Additionally affected by neurological conditions and disorders, adult neurogenesis is severely impacted by inflammation [174]. For instance, neuroinflammation has been shown to inhibit neurogenesis in the adult hippocampus; neurogenesis may be restored if inflammation is blocked [159, 175]. Adult mice kept on a protracted high-fat diet (HFD) exhibit markedly reduced neurogenesis in the hypothalamus which may also be due to neuroinflammatory reactions generated by the HFD [176, 177]. Contrarily, short-term HFD intake can result in an increase in hypothalamic neurogenesis, which is most likely an adaptive response of the hypothalamus to offset the detrimental effects of HFD feeding on energy balance [176]. The proliferation and differentiation of htNSCs generated from obese mice were shown to be hindered by Li et al., in their study. Such contortion resulted from the overproduction of inflammatory cytokines such TNF- and IL-1, which are known to potently activate IKK/NFκB and were created as a result of NFκB activation, leading to the activation of an inflammatory axis with a positive feed-forward loop [153]. IKK/NFκB activation significantly reduced in vitro htNSC survival, differentiation, and neurogenesis, while IKK/NFκB pathway inhibition increased htNSC survival, differentiation, and neurogenesis, providing additional and direct evidence of the harmful consequences of inflammation [153].

Even while it is established that hippocampal neurogenesis plays a crucial role in appropriate hippocampus function, learning, and memory, there was some scepticism about the report [178–180]. Two recent investigations, focusing in particular on the limited population of Pro-opiomelanocortin (POMC) neurons that play essential roles in regulating energy balance, showed that chronic HFD-induced obesity and

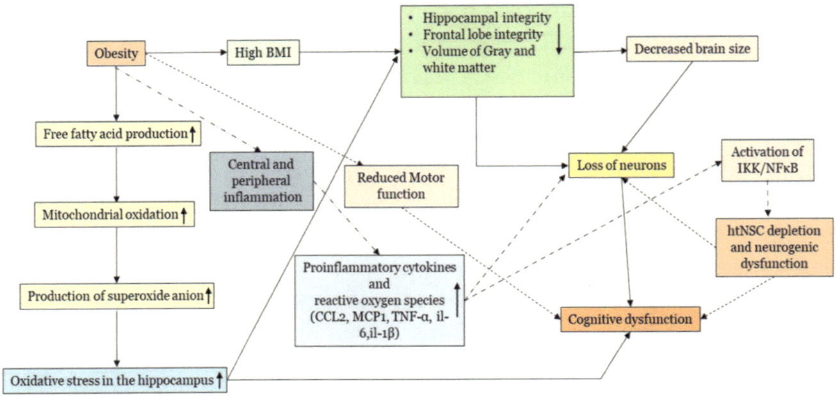

Figure 2.
Possible mechanism of obesity and cognitive dysfunction.

leptin deficit in mice resulted in a reduction in the adult NSC population and new neuron turnover [153]. Through the activation of multiple pro-inflammatory cascades, including the IKK/NFκB inflammatory axis, chronic HFD eating induces metabolic inflammation in the brain, particularly in the hypothalamus. Li et al. showed that chronic HFD eating in mice resulted in both htNSC depletion and neurogenic dysfunction linked to IKK/NFκB activation. The chronic consequences of metabolic dysfunctions, such as excessive calorie intake, glucose intolerance, insulin resistance, and obesity, were discovered in mice that had been genetically modified to have less NSCs in the MBH (**Figure 2**) [153].

7. Diet-induced obesity and synaptic plasticity dysfunction

The ability of the nervous system to dynamically modify its function in response to ongoing internal processes or outside events is referred to as the nervous system's plasticity [181]. It is a normal and important aspect of cognition as well as a key method through which the brain can heal after damage [182]. From fundamental physiological processes to integrated behavioural responses, plasticity can be understood and defined at many distinct levels of function [183, 184]. The physical morphology of synapses is related to structural plasticity [185]. Recent research has indicated that the HFD diet, which contains between 47 and 70% fat, has an impact on the brain's cognitive function [186–194]. According to this research, HFD causes negative consequences in various brain regions, including the hippocampus, via activating signalling pathways [195, 196]. HFD may have deleterious effects on memory and mood because it alters the systems that control synaptic transmission and the production of proteins associated with plasticity. HFD also causes obesity, which has an impact on the cellular and molecular mechanisms underlying synaptic plasticity in the brain, which impacts learning, memory, and mood. HFD also impaired brain-derived neurotrophic factors (BDNF), and amyloid precursor protein (APP) in the hippocampus.

7.1 Effects of obesity on BDNF

Neuroinflammation in the brain is a significant contributor to the development of neurodegenerative diseases. BDNF has the ability to regulate it [197]. This protein is required for the proper functional development of brain structures as well as the development and retention of synaptic transmission [198]. In addition to its conventional neurotrophic roles, BDNF also seems to have neuroprotective properties against a number of brain traumas, including as ischemia, traumatic brain injuries, and Alzheimer's disease [199]. It also significantly contributes to the metabolism of energy by reducing food intake, limiting weight gain, and enhancing locomotion following intracerebroventricular injection [183, 200]. Through molecules like synapsin I and growth-associated protein 43, BDNF can control neural plasticity [201, 202]. Synapsin I promotes BDNF modulation of synaptic vesicle exocytosis of neurotransmitters in addition to stimulating axonal growth and supporting synaptic connections [203]. It has been demonstrated that BDNF activation results in synapsin I phosphorylation [204, 205]. According to studies HFD consumption impairs hippocampus synaptic plasticity and cognitive capacities by regulating BDNF expression [206–209]. Other research has shown that HFD raises brain oxidative stress, which stimulates neuroinflammation and lowers levels of BDNF [186, 210]. After 4 months of HFD ingestion in mice, decreased levels of the basic synaptic proteins SNAP-25 and post-synaptic density (PSD)-95 may increase the brain's vulnerability to the negative effects of HFD [186].

7.2 Effects of obesity on APP

The biology of APP may have a role in the association between obesity and cognitive performance [211]. APP can be converted into the two peptides Ab1-40 and Ab1-42 by the brain's neurons, where it is mostly synthesised [212]. Amyloid plaques, a component of AD, are produced when both types of peptides are together [213]. Recent research suggests that the pathophysiology of obesity may also be influenced by APP expression or function [214]. The expression of APP in adipocyte cell lines and adipose tissue has been documented [215, 216]. More significantly, obese people have elevated plasma levels of adipose APP and Ab1-40 [216, 217]. Studies have shown that greater cholesterol levels induce higher amounts of amyloid- in both AD-transgenic and low-density lipoprotein receptor-deficient animals after 8 weeks of diet-dependent obesity in mice [214, 218, 219]. The APP expression or function modifications may be coordinated between several tissue types [214]. In contrast to visceral and subcutaneous fat, one study demonstrated variations in APP expression in brain cells [193]. Inflammation, macrophage and adipocyte phenotype, and macrophage and adipocyte culture phenotype were examined for comparison with the in vivo changes [193].

Another study discovered that feeding mice a very high-fat diet (HFD) for 5 weeks lowered the amounts of the cytoskeleton-associated protein (Arc), which controls baseline activity, in the cerebral cortex and hippocampus. The latter mice developed brain insulin resistance, and acute insulin stimulation reduced phosphatidylinositol 3-kinase (PI3K)/protein kinase B/p70 ribosomal S6 kinase pathway activity, which in turn reduced activation of Arc protein expression [193].

7.3 Effects of obesity on microglia

In addition to driving the inflammatory response in response to various stimuli, microglial cells also regularly maintain neurotrophic connections by remodelling and optimising synapses [220]. Microglia are said to react to neuroinflammation by releasing several kinds of macrovesicles [221]. For instance, when lipopolysaccharide activates BV2 microglial cells, the pro-inflammatory cytokines tumour necrosis factor and interleukin-6 are released [222]. Immature dendritic spine pattern in CA1 diIlabeled neurons, which showed decreased neurogenic ability and lower levels of the scaffold protein Shank 2, suggest impaired connection following an HFD (60% fat) [223]. The medial prefrontal cortex, a part of the brain crucial for cognitive flexibility, exhibits abnormalities in microglial morphology, synapse loss, and cognitive deficits in early-stage obese rats [189]. Additionally, it enhances synaptosome internalisation and microglial activation [191]. Mice given a 60% HFD were found to have fewer dendritic spines, higher levels of microglial activation, and higher levels of synaptic profiles within the microglia. Additionally, transgenic and pharmaceutical techniques that block microglial activation shield obese animals from cognitive deterioration and dendritic spine loss. Additionally, pharmaceutical reduction of microglia's phagocytic activity has been found to be adequate to stop cognitive decline [224].

7.4 The role of insulin receptors in memory

A crucial part of controlling body metabolism is insulin. However, insulin modifies neural activity, strengthening synaptic connections and increasing memory function [225–227]. Insulin is known to have profound effects on neurotransmission [228]. PSD fractions contain insulin receptors, which are heavily concentrated in synaptosomes [229]. The scaffolding proteins shank and PSD-95 may also interact with them through insulin receptor tyrosine kinase substrate IRSp53, which is colocalized with synaptophysin and synapsin 1 [230, 231]. Neurites are promoted by insulin, catecholamine release and uptake is regulated, ligand-gated ion channel trafficking is controlled, gamma-aminobutyric acid, N-methyl-d-aspartic acid (NMDA) and AMPA receptors are expressed and localised, and NMDA and PI3K-Akt are involved in modulating synaptic plasticity [232]. There has been significant evidence that insulin resistance and the metabolic syndrome may cause cognitive impairments through mechanisms such as IPMK-mTOR/Akt, synapto-dendritic molecular neuroanatomy, and spatial working memory [233]. In mice, diets high in fat lead to insulin resistance in the cerebral cortex and hypothalamus. Several animal models have shown that insulin resistance affects cognition-related circuitry and neurotransmission [187, 226].

Studies in animals have found reduced dendritic spines in CA1 as well as impairments in long-term memory associated with HFD feeding [191, 234, 235]. Many different parts of the brain can be negatively impacted by alterations in glucose homeostasis, but the hippocampus is particularly susceptible to them [236–238]. According to research by Strahan et al., rats fed a high-fat, high-glucose diet for 8 months showed significant impairments in their hippocampal dendritic spine density, spatial learning ability, and LTP at Schaffer collateral-CA1 synapses [239]. In addition, high-fat, high-glucose-fed animals showed a reduction in BDNF levels in the hippocampus compared with controls. They suggested that the changes could be due to peripheral insulin resistance, or that some components of the diet may directly affect brain health and hippocampal plasticity. Further evidence suggests that the DG of rats fed HFD exhibit impaired stimulus-evoked LTP [240]. HFD feeding leads to a change in the expression of protein-coding genes in the cortex, but studies have not explored alterations in non-coding RNAs. The HFD feeding of mice led to changes in both coding and non-coding RNA expression in the brain cortex, according to a study by Yoon and colleagues. According to these researchers, consuming HFD for 8 weeks causes a decrease in the expression of genes linked to synaptogenesis and neurotransmitter release [241]. In the hippocampus of animals receiving HFD, Arnold, and colleagues likewise found that PSD-95 expression was downregulated [187]. Interesting investigations have found that animals given the HFD have less neurogenesis in their dentate gyrus [242]. Thus, it is clear that HFD may significantly modify the expression of many genes linked to these processes, which may have a negative impact on brain morphology and synaptic plasticity.

8. Conclusion

Obesity is a serious public health problem that is increasing an proportions with serious health and societal problems. It mostly affects cognition through changing the structures and operations of the brain. Brain structure, leptin/insulin dysregulation, oxidative stress, cerebrovascular function, blood-brain barrier, and inflammation are all impacted by obesity and contribute to the decline in cognitive performance. Inhibition of neurogenesis is thought to be caused by neuroinflammation, which can be brought on by a variety of internal or external factors, including ER and oxidative stress, as well as, overnutrition-induced metabolic inflammation, and autophagic defects. These factors are all connected to the activation of the central IKK/NF-B inflammatory signalling cascade, which can result in a vicious inflammatory cycle that accelerates ageing, neurodegeneration, and cognitive decline.

Author details

Amina Khatun[1], Surendra Patra[1], Kuntal Ghosh[1], Shrabani Pradhan[2] and Sudipta Chakrabarti[1*]

1 Department of Biological Sciences, Midnapore City College, Kuturiya, Bhadutala, Paschim Medinipur, West Bengal, India

2 Department of Paramedical and Allied Health Science, Midnapore City College, Kuturiya, Bhadutala, Paschim Medinipur, West Bengal, India

*Address all correspondence to: sudiptadna@gmail.com

References

[1] Mcardle MA, Finucane OM, Connaughton RM, Mcmorrow AM, Roche HM. Mechanisms of obesity-induced inflammation and insulin resistance: Insights into the emerging role of nutritional strategies. Frontiers in Endocrinology. 2013;**4**:52

[2] Kant AK. Dietary patterns and health outcomes. Journal of the American Dietetic Association. 2004;**104**:615-635

[3] Mcewen BS, Morrison JH. The brain on stress: Vulnerability and plasticity of the prefrontal cortex over the life course. Neuron. 2013;**79**:16-29

[4] Schwartz MW, Porte D Jr. Diabetes, obesity, and the brain. Science. 2005;**307**:375-379

[5] Organization WH. Obesity and overweight. Fact sheet N 311. 2012. Available from: http://www.who.int/mediacentre/factsheets/fs311/en/

[6] Klöting N, Blüher M. Adipocyte dysfunction, inflammation and metabolic syndrome. Reviews in Endocrine and Metabolic Disorders. 2014;**15**:277-287

[7] Stillman CM, Weinstein AM, Marsland AL, Gianaros PJ, Erickson KI. Body–brain connections: The effects of obesity and behavioral interventions on neurocognitive aging. Frontiers in Aging Neuroscience. 2017;**9**:115

[8] Timper K, Brüning JC. Hypothalamic circuits regulating appetite and energy homeostasis: Pathways to obesity. Disease Models & Mechanisms. 2017;**10**:679-689

[9] Do'Brien P, Hinder LM, Callaghan BC, Feldman EL. Neurological consequences of obesity. The Lancet Neurology. 2017;**16**:465-477

[10] Dienel GA. Fueling and imaging brain activation. ASN Neuro. 2012;**4** AN20120021

[11] Bordone MP, Salman MM, Titus HE, Amini E, Andersen JV, Chakraborti B, et al. The energetic brain–a review from students to students. Journal of Neurochemistry. 2019;**151**:139-165

[12] Gomez-Pinilla F, Tyagi E. Diet and cognition: Interplay between cell metabolism and neuronal plasticity. Current Opinion in Clinical Nutrition and Metabolic Care. 2013;**16**:726

[13] Mattson MP. Energy intake and exercise as determinants of brain health and vulnerability to injury and disease. Cell Metabolism. 2012;**16**:706-722

[14] Greenwood CE, Winocur G. High-fat diets, insulin resistance and declining cognitive function. Neurobiology of Aging. 2005;**26**:42-45

[15] Molteni R, Barnard R, Ying Z, Roberts C, Gomez-Pinilla F. A high-fat, refined sugar diet reduces hippocampal brain-derived neurotrophic factor, neuronal plasticity, and learning. Neuroscience. 2002;**112**:803-814

[16] Bayer-Carter JL, Green PS, Montine TJ, Vanfossen B, Baker LD, Watson GS, et al. Diet intervention and cerebrospinal fluid biomarkers in amnestic mild cognitive impairment. Archives of Neurology. 2011;**68**:743-752

[17] Edwards LM, Murray AJ, Holloway CJ, Carter EE, Kemp GJ, Codreanu I, et al. Short-term consumption of a high-fat diet impairs

whole-body efficiency and cognitive function in sedentary men. The FASEB Journal. 2011;**25**:1088-1096

[18] Eskelinen MH, Ngandu T, Helkala EL, Tuomilehto J, Nissinen A, Soininen H, et al. Fat intake at midlife and cognitive impairment later in life: A population-based CAIDE study. International Journal of Geriatric Psychiatry: A Journal of the Psychiatry of Late Life and Allied Sciences. 2008;**23**:741-747

[19] Mccann JC, Ames BN. Is docosahexaenoic acid, an n− 3 long-chain polyunsaturated fatty acid, required for development of normal brain function? An overview of evidence from cognitive and behavioral tests in humans and animals. The American Journal of Clinical Nutrition. 2005;**82**:281-295

[20] Wu A, Ying Z, Gomez-Pinilla F. Omega-3 fatty acids supplementation restores mechanisms that maintain brain homeostasis in traumatic brain injury. Journal of Neurotrauma. 2007;**24**:1587-1595

[21] Crescenzo R, Bianco F, Mazzoli A, Giacco A, Cancelliere R, Di Fabio G, et al. Fat quality influences the obesogenic effect of high fat diets. Nutrients. 2015;7:9475-9491

[22] Kraegen EW, Clark PW, Jenkins AB, Daley EA, Chisholm DJ, Storlien LH. Development of muscle insulin resistance after liver insulin resistance in high-fat–fed rats. Diabetes. 1991;**40**:1397-1403

[23] Siri-Tarino PW, Sun Q, Hu FB, Krauss RM. Saturated fat, carbohydrate, and cardiovascular disease. The American Journal of Clinical Nutrition. 2010;**91**:502-509

[24] Biessels GJ, Despa F. Cognitive decline and dementia in diabetes mellitus: Mechanisms and clinical implications. Nature Reviews Endocrinology. 2018;**14**:591-604

[25] Chatterjee S, Peters SA, Woodward M, Mejia Arango S, Batty GD, Beckett N, et al. Type 2 diabetes as a risk factor for dementia in women compared with men: A pooled analysis of 2.3 million people comprising more than 100,000 cases of dementia. Diabetes Care. 2016;**39**:300-307

[26] Crane PK, Walker R, Hubbard RA, Li G, Nathan DM, Zheng H, et al. Glucose levels and risk of dementia. New England Journal of Medicine. 2013;**369**:540-548

[27] de Felice FG, Lourenco MV, Ferreira ST. How does brain insulin resistance develop in Alzheimer's disease? Alzheimer's & Dementia. 2014;**10**:S26-S32

[28] Balistreri CR, Caruso C, Candore G. The role of adipose tissue and adipokines in obesity-related inflammatory diseases. Mediators of Inflammation. 2010;**2010**

[29] Hill JO, Wyatt HR, Peters JC. Energy balance and obesity. Circulation. 2012;**126**:126-132

[30] de Souza RJ, Bray GA, Carey VJ, Hall KD, Leboff MS, Loria CM, et al. Effects of 4 weight-loss diets differing in fat, protein, and carbohydrate on fat mass, lean mass, visceral adipose tissue, and hepatic fat: Results from the POUNDS LOST trial. The American Journal of Clinical Nutrition. 2012;**95**:614-625

[31] Fall T, Mendelson M, Speliotes EK. Recent advances in human genetics and epigenetics of adiposity: Pathway to precision medicine? Gastroenterology. 2017;**152**:1695-1706

[32] Locke AE, Kahali B, Berndt SI, Justice AE, Pers TH, Day FR, et al. Genetic studies of body mass index yield new insights for obesity biology. Nature. 2015;**518**:197-206

[33] Angulo M, Butler M, Cataletto M. Prader-Willi syndrome: A review of clinical, genetic, and endocrine findings. Journal of Endocrinological Investigation. 2015;**38**:1249-1263

[34] Albuquerque D, Nóbrega C, Manco L, Padez C. The contribution of genetics and environment to obesity. British Medical Bulletin. 2017;**123**:159-173

[35] Schwartz MW, Seeley RJ, Zeltser LM, DRewnowski A, Ravussin E, Redman LM, et al. Obesity pathogenesis: An endocrine society scientific statement. Endocrine Reviews. 2017;**38**:267-296

[36] Hall KD, Guo J. Obesity energetics: Body weight regulation and the effects of diet composition. Gastroenterology. 2017;**152**:1718-1727. e3

[37] Rosen ED, Spiegelman BM. What we talk about when we talk about fat. Cell. 2014;**156**:20-44

[38] Kalupahana NS, Moustaid-Moussa N. The renin-angiotensin system: A link between obesity, inflammation and insulin resistance. Obesity Reviews. 2012;**13**:136-149

[39] Bartness TJ, Shrestha Y, Vaughan C, Schwartz G, Song C. Sensory and sympathetic nervous system control of white adipose tissue lipolysis. Molecular and Cellular Endocrinology. 2010;**318**:34-43

[40] Smith MM, Minson CT. Obesity and adipokines: Effects on sympathetic overactivity. The Journal of Physiology. 2012;**590**:1787-1801

[41] Brooks SJ, Benedict C, Burgos J, Kempton M, Kullberg J, Nordenskjöld R, et al. Late-life obesity is associated with smaller global and regional gray matter volumes: A voxel-based morphometric study. International Journal of Obesity. 2013;**37**:230-236

[42] Gazdzinski S, Kornak J, Weiner MW, Meyerhoff DJ. Body mass index and magnetic resonance markers of brain integrity in adults. Annals of Neurology. 2008;**63**:652-657

[43] Pannacciulli N, Del Parigi A, Chen K, Le DSN, Reiman EM, Tataranni PA. Brain abnormalities in human obesity: A voxel-based morphometric study. NeuroImage. 2006;**31**:1419-1425

[44] Raji CA, Ho AJ, Parikshak NN, Becker JT, Lopez OL, Kuller LH, et al. Brain structure and obesity. Human Brain Mapping. 2010;**31**:353-364

[45] Herrmann MJ, Tesar AK, Beier J, Berg M, Warrings B. Grey matter alterations in obesity: A meta-analysis of whole-brain studies. Obesity Reviews. 2019;**20**:464-471

[46] Haltia LT, Viljanen A, Parkkola R, Kemppainen N, Rinne JO, Nuutila P, et al. Brain white matter expansion in human obesity and the recovering effect of dieting. The Journal of Clinical Endocrinology & Metabolism. 2007;**92**:3278-3284

[47] Jauch-Chara K, Binkofski F, Loebig M, Reetz K, Jahn G, Melchert UH, et al. Blunted brain energy consumption relates to insula atrophy and impaired glucose tolerance in obesity. Diabetes. 2015;**64**:2082-2091

[48] Karlsson HK, Tuulari JJ, Hirvonen J, Lepomäki V, Parkkola R, Hiltunen J, et al. Obesity is associated with white matter atrophy: A combined diffusion tensor

imaging and voxel-based morphometric study. Obesity. 2013;**21**:2530-2537

[49] Mathar D, Horstmann A, Pleger B, Villringer A, Neumann J. Is it worth the effort? Novel insights into obesity-associated alterations in cost-benefit decision-making. Frontiers in Behavioral Neuroscience. 2016;**9**:360

[50] Shott ME, Cornier M-A, Mittal VA, Pryor TL, Orr JM, Brown MS, et al. Orbitofrontal cortex volume and brain reward response in obesity. International Journal of Obesity. 2015;**39**:214-221

[51] Tuulari JJ, Karlsson HK, Antikainen O, Hirvonen J, Pham T, Salminen P, et al. Bariatric surgery induces white and grey matter density recovery in the morbidly obese: A voxel-based morphometric study. Human Brain Mapping. 2016;**37**:3745-3756

[52] Wang H, Wen B, Cheng J, Li H. Brain structural differences between normal and obese adults and their links with lack of perseverance, negative urgency, and sensation seeking. Scientific Reports. 2017;7:1-7

[53] Zhang B, Tian X, Tian D, Wang J, Wang Q, Yu C, et al. Altered regional gray matter volume in obese men: A structural MRI study. Frontiers in Psychology. 2017;**8**:125

[54] Kurth F, Levitt JG, Phillips OR, Luders E, Woods RP, Mazziotta JC, et al. Relationships between gray matter, body mass index, and waist circumference in healthy adults. Human Brain Mapping. 2013;**34**:1737-1746

[55] García-García I, Michaud A, Dadar M, Zeighami Y, Neseliler S, Collins DL, et al. Neuroanatomical differences in obesity: Meta-analytic findings and their validation in an independent dataset. International Journal of Obesity. 2019;**43**:943-951

[56] Yokum S, Ng J, Stice E. Relation of regional gray and white matter volumes to current BMI and future increases in BMI: A prospective MRI study. International Journal of Obesity. 2012;**36**:656-664

[57] He Q, Chen C, Dong Q, Xue G, Chen C, Lu Z-L, et al. Gray and white matter structures in the midcingulate cortex region contribute to body mass index in Chinese young adults. Brain Structure and Function. 2015;**220**:319-329

[58] Papageorgiou I, Astrakas LG, Xydis V, Alexiou GA, Bargiotas P, Tzarouchi L, et al. Abnormalities of brain neural circuits related to obesity: A diffusion tensor imaging study. Magnetic Resonance Imaging. 2017;**37**:116-121

[59] Repple J, Opel N, Meinert S, Redlich R, Hahn T, Winter NR, et al. Elevated body-mass index is associated with reduced white matter integrity in two large independent cohorts. Psychoneuroendocrinology. 2018;**91**:179-185

[60] Cai D. Neuroinflammation and neurodegeneration in overnutrition-induced diseases. Trends in Endocrinology & Metabolism. 2013;**24**:40-47

[61] Kullmann S, Callaghan MF, Heni M, Weiskopf N, Scheffler K, Häring H-U, et al. Specific white matter tissue microstructure changes associated with obesity. NeuroImage. 2016;**125**:36-44

[62] Kim A-Y, Shim J-H, Choi HJ, Baek H-M. Comparison of volumetric and shape changes of subcortical structures based on 3-dimensional image between obesity and normal-weighted subjects

using 3.0 T MRI. Journal of Clinical Neuroscience. 2020;**73**:280-287

[63] Yau PL, Kang EH, Javier DC, Convit A. Preliminary evidence of cognitive and brain abnormalities in uncomplicated adolescent obesity. Obesity. 2014;**22**:1865-1871

[64] Ryan JP, Fine DF, Rosano C. Type 2 diabetes and cognitive impairment: Contributions from neuroimaging. Journal of Geriatric Psychiatry and Neurology. 2014;**27**:47-55

[65] Van Opstal A, Wijngaarden M, Van der Grond J, Pijl H. Changes in brain activity after weight loss. Obesity Science & Practice. 2019;**5**:459-467

[66] Opel N, Thalamuthu A, Milaneschi Y, Grotegerd D, Flint C, Leenings R, et al. Brain structural abnormalities in obesity: Relation to age, genetic risk, and common psychiatric disorders. Molecular Psychiatry. 2021;**26**:4839-4852

[67] Wang C, Chan JS, Ren L, Yan JH. Obesity reduces cognitive and motor functions across the lifespan. Neural Plasticity. 2016;**2016**

[68] Hess LM. Chemotherapy-related change in cognitive function: A conceptual model. 1969;**34**(5):981-994

[69] Bolzenius JD, Laidlaw DH, Cabeen RP, Conturo TE, Mcmichael AR, Lane EM, et al. Brain structure and cognitive correlates of body mass index in healthy older adults. Behavioural Brain Research. 2015;**278**:342-347

[70] Volkow ND, Wang GJ, Telang F, Fowler JS, Goldstein RZ, Alia-Klein N, et al. Inverse association between BMI and prefrontal metabolic activity in healthy adults. Obesity. 2009;**17**:60-65

[71] Walther K, Birdsill AC, Glisky EL, Ryan L. Structural brain differences and cognitive functioning related to body mass index in older females. Human Brain Mapping. 2010;**31**:1052-1064

[72] Whitmer RA, Gunderson EP, Barrett-Connor E, Quesenberry CP, Yaffe K. Obesity in middle age and future risk of dementia: A 27 year longitudinal population based study. BMJ. 2005;**330**:1360

[73] Van den Berg E, Kloppenborg RP, Kessels RP, Kappelle LJ, Biessels GJ. Type 2 diabetes mellitus, hypertension, dyslipidemia and obesity: A systematic comparison of their impact on cognition. Biochimica et Biophysica Acta (BBA)-Molecular Basis of Disease. 2009;**1792**:470-481

[74] Cserjési R, Molnár D, Luminet O, Lénárd L. Is there any relationship between obesity and mental flexibility in children? Appetite. 2007;**49**:675-678

[75] Davis CL, Tomporowski PD, Mcdowell JE, Austin BP, Miller PH, Yanasak NE, et al. Exercise improves executive function and achievement and alters brain activation in overweight children: A randomized, controlled trial. Health Psychology. 2011;**30**:91

[76] Jansen P, Schmelter A, Kasten L, Heil M. Impaired mental rotation performance in overweight children. Appetite. 2011;**56**:766-769

[77] Kamijo K, Khan NA, Pontifex MB, Scudder MR, Drollette ES, Raine LB, et al. The relation of adiposity to cognitive control and scholastic achievement in preadolescent children. Obesity. 2012;**20**:2406-2411

[78] Verdejo-García A, Pérez-Expósito M, Schmidt-Río-Valle J, Fernández-Serrano MJ, Cruz F, Pérez-García M, et al. Selective

alterations within executive functions in adolescents with excess weight. Obesity. 2010;**18**:1572-1578

[79] Lokken KL, Boeka AG, Austin HM, Gunstad J, Harmon CM. Evidence of executive dysfunction in extremely obese adolescents: A pilot study. Surgery for Obesity and Related Diseases. 2009;**5**:547-552

[80] Schwartz DH, Leonard G, Perron M, Richer L, Syme C, Veillette S, et al. Visceral fat is associated with lower executive functioning in adolescents. International Journal of Obesity. 2013;**37**:1336-1343

[81] Mond J, Stich H, Hay P, Krämer A, Baune B. Associations between obesity and developmental functioning in pre-school children: A population-based study. International Journal of Obesity. 2007;**31**:1068-1073

[82] Slining M, Adair LS, Goldman BD, Borja JB, Bentley M. Infant overweight is associated with delayed motor development. The Journal of Pediatrics. 2010;**157**:20-25. e1

[83] Southall JE, Okely AD, Steele JR. Actual and perceived physical competence in overweight and nonoverweight children. Pediatric Exercise Science. 2004;**16**:15-24

[84] Poulsen AA, Desha L, Ziviani J, Griffiths L, Heaslop A, Khan A, et al. Fundamental movement skills and self-concept of children who are overweight. International Journal of Pediatric Obesity. 2011;**6**:e464-e471

[85] Roberts D, Veneri D, Decker R, Gannotti M. Weight status and gross motor skill in kindergarten children. Pediatric Physical Therapy. 2012;**24**:353-360

[86] Krombholz H. Motor and cognitive performance of overweight preschool children. Perceptual and Motor Skills. 2013;**116**:40-57

[87] Gentier I, D'hondt E, Shultz S, Deforche B, Augustijn M, Hoorne S, et al. Fine and gross motor skills differ between healthy-weight and obese children. Research in Developmental Disabilities. 2013;**34**:4043-4051

[88] Garbarino VR, Orr ME, Rodriguez KA, Buffenstein R. Mechanisms of oxidative stress resistance in the brain: Lessons learned from hypoxia tolerant extremophilic vertebrates. Archives of Biochemistry and Biophysics. 2015;**576**:8-16

[89] Verdile G, Keane KN, Cruzat VF, Medic S, Sabale M, Rowles J, et al. Inflammation and oxidative stress: The molecular connectivity between insulin resistance, obesity, and Alzheimer's disease. Mediators of Inflammation. 2015;**2015**

[90] Tan BL, Norhaizan ME. Effect of high-fat diets on oxidative stress, cellular inflammatory response and cognitive function. Nutrients. 2019;**11**:2579

[91] Tangvarasittichai S. Oxidative stress, insulin resistance, dyslipidemia and type 2 diabetes mellitus. World Journal of Diabetes. 2015;**6**:456

[92] Pessayre D, Mansouri A, Fromenty B. V. Mitochondrial dysfunction in steatohepatitis. American Journal of Physiology-Gastrointestinal and Liver Physiology. 2002;**282**:G193-G199

[93] Matsuzawa-Nagata N, Takamura T, Ando H, Nakamura S, Kurita S, Misu H, et al. Increased oxidative stress precedes the onset of high-fat diet–induced insulin resistance and obesity. Metabolism. 2008;**57**:1071-1077

[94] Le Lay S, Simard G, Martinez MC, Andriantsitohaina R. Oxidative stress and metabolic pathologies: From an adipocentric point of view. Oxidative Medicine and Cellular Longevity. 2014;**2014**

[95] Head E. Oxidative damage and cognitive dysfunction: Antioxidant treatments to promote healthy brain aging. Neurochemical Research. 2009;**34**:670-678

[96] Perry G, Moreira PI, Santos MS, Oliveira CR, Shenk JC, Nunomura A, et al. Alzheimer disease and the role of free radicals in the pathogenesis of the disease. CNS & Neurological Disorders-Drug Targets (Formerly Current Drug Targets-CNS & Neurological Disorders). 2008;**7**:3-10

[97] Perry G, Nunomura A, Hirai K, Zhu X, Prez M, Avila J, et al. Is oxidative damage the fundamental pathogenic mechanism of Alzheimer's and other neurodegenerative diseases? Free Radical Biology and Medicine. 2002;**33**:1475-1479

[98] Su B, Wang X, Nunomura A, Moreira PI, Lee H-G, Perry G, et al. Oxidative stress signaling in Alzheimer's disease. Current Alzheimer Research. 2008;**5**:525-532

[99] Kumar A, Jaggi AS, Sodhi RK, Singh N. Silymarin ameliorates memory deficits and neuropathological changes in mouse model of high-fat-diet-induced experimental dementia. Naunyn-Schmiedeberg's Archives of Pharmacology. 2014;**387**:777-787

[100] Liu Y, Fu X, Lan N, Li S, Zhang J, Wang S, et al. Luteolin protects against high fat diet-induced cognitive deficits in obesity mice. Behavioural Brain Research. 2014;**267**:178-188

[101] Lu J, Wu D-M, Zheng Z-H, Zheng Y-L, Hu B, Zhang Z-F. Troxerutin protects against high cholesterol-induced cognitive deficits in mice. Brain. 2011;**134**:783-797

[102] Pintana H, Apaijai N, Chattipakorn N, Chattipakorn SC. DPP-4 inhibitors improve cognition and brain mitochondrial function of insulin-resistant rats. The Journal of Endocrinology. 2013;**218**:1-11

[103] Pintana H, Apaijai N, Pratchayasakul W, Chattipakorn N, Chattipakorn SC. Effects of metformin on learning and memory behaviors and brain mitochondrial functions in high fat diet induced insulin resistant rats. Life Sciences. 2012;**91**:409-414

[104] Sodhi RK, Singh N. Liver X receptor agonist T0901317 reduces neuropathological changes and improves memory in mouse models of experimental dementia. European Journal of Pharmacology. 2014;**732**:50-59

[105] de Oliveira MR, Rocha RFD, Stertz L, Fries GR, de Oliveira DL, Kapczinski F, et al. Total and mitochondrial nitrosative stress, decreased brain-derived neurotrophic factor (BDNF) levels and glutamate uptake, and evidence of endoplasmic reticulum stress in the hippocampus of vitamin A-treated rats. Neurochemical Research. 2011;**36**:506-517

[106] Evans JL, Goldfine ID, Maddux BA, Grodsky GM. Are oxidative stress–activated signaling pathways mediators of insulin resistance and β-cell dysfunction? Diabetes. 2003;**52**:1-8

[107] Farr SA, Yamada KA, Butterfield DA, Abdul HM, Xu L, Miller NE, et al. Obesity and hypertriglyceridemia produce cognitive impairment. Endocrinology. 2008;**149**:2628-2636

[108] Stranahan AM, Cutler RG, Button C, Telljohann R, Mattson MP. Diet-induced elevations in serum cholesterol are associated with alterations in hippocampal lipid metabolism and increased oxidative stress. Journal of Neurochemistry. 2011;**118**:611-615

[109] Alzoubi KH, Khabour OF, Salah HA, Hasan Z. Vitamin E prevents high-fat high-carbohydrates diet-induced memory impairment: The role of oxidative stress. Physiology & Behavior. 2013;**119**:72-78

[110] Xia S-F, Xie Z-X, Qiao Y, Li L-R, Cheng X-R, Duan X-M, et al. Salvianolic acid B counteracts cognitive decline triggered by oxidative stress in mice fed with high-fat diets. Journal of Functional Foods. 2014;**11**:278-292

[111] O'shea JJ, Murray PJ. Cytokine signaling modules in inflammatory responses. Immunity. 2008;**28**:477-487

[112] Lumeng CN, Bodzin JL, Saltiel AR. Obesity induces a phenotypic switch in adipose tissue macrophage polarization. The Journal of Clinical Investigation. 2007;**117**:175-184

[113] Zeyda M, Stulnig TM. Adipose tissue macrophages. Immunology Letters. 2007;**112**:61-67

[114] Poltavets AS, Vishnyakova PA, Elchaninov AV, Sukhikh GT, Fatkhudinov TK. Macrophage modification strategies for efficient cell therapy. Cell. 2020;**9**:1535

[115] Hahm JR, Jo MH, Ullah R, Kim MW, Kim MO. Metabolic stress alters antioxidant systems, suppresses the adiponectin receptor 1 and induces Alzheimer's like pathology in mice brain. Cell. 2020;**9**:249

[116] Nguyen JC, Killcross AS, Jenkins TA. Obesity and cognitive decline: Role of inflammation and vascular changes. Frontiers in Neuroscience. 2014;**8**:375

[117] Cinti S, Mitchell G, Barbatelli G, Murano I, Ceresi E, Faloia E, et al. Adipocyte death defines macrophage localization and function in adipose tissue of obese mice and humans. Journal of Lipid Research. 2005;**46**:2347-2355

[118] Mosser DM, Edwards JP. Exploring the full spectrum of macrophage activation. Nature Reviews Immunology. 2008;**8**:958-969

[119] Bastard J-P, Maachi M, Lagathu C, Kim MJ, Caron M, Vidal H, et al. Recent advances in the relationship between obesity, inflammation, and insulin resistance. European Cytokine Network. 2006;**17**:4-12

[120] Agustí A, García-Pardo MP, López-Almela I, Campillo I, Maes M, Romaní-Pérez M, et al. Interplay between the gut-brain axis, obesity and cognitive function. Frontiers in Neuroscience. 2018;**12**:155

[121] Valdes AM, Walter J, Segal E, Spector TD. Role of the gut microbiota in nutrition and health. BMJ. 2018;**361**

[122] Baothman OA, Zamzami MA, Taher I, Abubaker J, Abu-Farha M. The role of gut microbiota in the development of obesity and diabetes. Lipids in Health and Disease. 2016;**15**:1-8

[123] Kim Y-G, Udayanga KGS, Totsuka N, Weinberg JB, Núñez G, Shibuya A. Gut dysbiosis promotes M2 macrophage polarization and allergic airway inflammation via fungi-induced PGE2. Cell Host & Microbe. 2014;**15**:95-102

[124] Slyepchenko A, Maes M, Jacka FN, Köhler CA, Barichello T, Mcintyre RS, et al. Gut microbiota,

bacterial translocation, and interactions with diet: Pathophysiological links between major depressive disorder and non-communicable medical comorbidities. Psychotherapy and Psychosomatics. 2017;**86**:31-46

[125] Guillemot-Legris O, Muccioli GG. Obesity-induced neuroinflammation: Beyond the hypothalamus. Trends in Neurosciences. 2017;**40**:237-253

[126] Novo AM, Batista S. Multiple sclerosis: Implications of obesity in neuroinflammation. Obesity and Brain Function. 2017:191-210

[127] Segarra M, Aburto MR, Acker-Palmer A. Blood–brain barrier dynamics to maintain brain homeostasis. Trends in Neurosciences. 2021;**44**:393-405

[128] Parimisetty A, Dorsemans A-C, Awada R, Ravanan P, Diotel N, LEfebvre D'Hellencourt, C. Secret talk between adipose tissue and central nervous system via secreted factors—An emerging frontier in the neurodegenerative research. Journal of Neuroinflammation. 2016;**13**:1-13

[129] Stolp H, Dziegielewska K. Role of developmental inflammation and blood–brain barrier dysfunction in neurodevelopmental and neurodegenerative diseases. Neuropathology and Applied Neurobiology. 2009;**35**:132-146

[130] Pugazhenthi S, Qin L, Reddy PH. Common neurodegenerative pathways in obesity, diabetes, and Alzheimer's disease. Biochimica et Biophysica Acta (BBA)-Molecular Basis of Disease. 2017;**1863**:1037-1045

[131] Spielman LJ, Little JP, Klegeris A. Inflammation and insulin/IGF-1 resistance as the possible link between obesity and neurodegeneration. Journal of Neuroimmunology. 2014;**273**:8-21

[132] Miller AA, Spencer SJ. Obesity and neuroinflammation: A pathway to cognitive impairment. Brain, Behavior, and Immunity. 2014;**42**:10-21

[133] Herradon G, Ramos-Alvarez MP, Gramage E. Connecting metainflammation and neuroinflammation through the PTN-MK-RPTPβ/ζ axis: Relevance in therapeutic development. Frontiers in Pharmacology. 2019;**10**:377

[134] Ajami B, Bennett JL, Krieger C, Tetzlaff W, Rossi F. Local self-renewal can sustain CNS microglia maintenance and function throughout adult life. Nature Neuroscience. 2007;**10**:1538-1543

[135] Keshk WA, Ibrahim MA, Shalaby SM, Zalat ZA, Elseady WS. Redox status, inflammation, necroptosis and inflammasome as indispensable contributors to high fat diet (HFD)-induced neurodegeneration; effect of N-acetylcysteine (NAC). Archives of Biochemistry and Biophysics. 2020;**680**:108227

[136] Daulatzai MA. Cerebral hypoperfusion and glucose hypometabolism: Key pathophysiological modulators promote neurodegeneration, cognitive impairment, and Alzheimer's disease. Journal of Neuroscience Research. 2017;**95**:943-972

[137] Dey A, Allen JN, Fraser JW, Snyder LM, Tian Y, Zhang L, et al. Neuroprotective role of the Ron receptor tyrosine kinase underlying central nervous system inflammation in health and disease. Frontiers in Immunology. 2018;**9**:513

[138] Fricker M, Tolkovsky AM, Borutaite V, Coleman M, Brown GC.

Neuronal cell death. Physiological Reviews. 2018;**98**:813-880

[139] Jan R. Understanding apoptosis and apoptotic pathways targeted cancer therapeutics. Advanced Pharmaceutical Bulletin. 2019;**9**:205

[140] Xu X, Lai Y, Hua Z-C. Apoptosis and apoptotic body: Disease message and therapeutic target potentials. Bioscience Reports. 2019;**39**

[141] Green DR, Llambi F. Cell death signaling. Cold Spring Harbor Perspectives in Biology. 2015;**7**:a006080

[142] Kumari A, Kumar P, Yadav A. Impact of physical activity on central nervous system, neurogenesis and brains aging. Journal for Reattach Therapy and Developmental Diversities. 2022;**5**:229-234

[143] Altman J. Are new neurons formed in the brains of adult mammals? Science. 1962;**135**:1127-1128

[144] Altman J, Das GD. Post-natal origin of microneurones in the rat brain. Nature. 1965;**207**:953-956

[145] Rakic P. Limits of neurogenesis in primates. Science. 1985;**227**:1054-1056

[146] Gould E, Reeves AJ, Fallah M, Tanapat P, Gross CG, Fuchs E. Hippocampal neurogenesis in adult Old World primates. Proceedings of the National Academy of Sciences. 1999b;**96**:5263-5267

[147] Kornack DR, Rakic P. Continuation of neurogenesis in the hippocampus of the adult macaque monkey. Proceedings of the National Academy of Sciences. 1999;**96**:5768-5773

[148] Cameron HA, Mckay R. Discussion point stem cells and neurogenesis in the adult brain. Current Opinion in Neurobiology. 1998;**8**:677-680

[149] Gage FH. Mammalian neural stem cells. Science. 2000;**287**:1433-1438

[150] Reynolds BA, Weiss S. Generation of neurons and astrocytes from isolated cells of the adult mammalian central nervous system. Science. 1992;**255**:1707-1710

[151] Alvarez-Buylla A, Lim DA. For the long run: Maintaining germinal niches in the adult brain. Neuron. 2004;**41**:683-686

[152] Emsley JG, Mitchell BD, Kempermann G, Macklis JD. Adult neurogenesis and repair of the adult CNS with neural progenitors, precursors, and stem cells. Progress in Neurobiology. 2005;**75**:321-341

[153] Li J, Tang Y, Cai D. IKKβ/NF-κB disrupts adult hypothalamic neural stem cells to mediate a neurodegenerative mechanism of dietary obesity and pre-diabetes. Nature Cell Biology. 2012;**14**:999-1012

[154] Song H-J, Stevens CF, Gage FH. Neural stem cells from adult hippocampus develop essential properties of functional CNS neurons. Nature Neuroscience. 2002;**5**:438-445

[155] Cai D. One Step from Prediabetes to Diabetes: Hypothalamic Inflammation? Oxford University Press; 2012

[156] Cai D, Liu T. Hypothalamic inflammation: A double-edged sword to nutritional diseases. Annals of the New York Academy of Sciences. 2011;**1243**:E1-E39

[157] Purkayastha S, Cai D. Disruption of neurogenesis by hypothalamic inflammation in obesity or aging.

Reviews in Endocrine and Metabolic Disorders. 2013;**14**:351-356

[158] Zhang G, Li J, Purkayastha S, Tang Y, Zhang H, Yin Y, et al. Hypothalamic programming of systemic ageing involving IKK-β, NF-κB and GnRH. Nature. 2013;**497**:211-216

[159] Ekdahl CT, Claasen J-H, Bonde S, Kokaia Z, Lindvall O. Inflammation is detrimental for neurogenesis in adult brain. Proceedings of the National Academy of Sciences. 2003;**100**:13632-13637

[160] Eikelenboom P, Veerhuis R, Scheper W, Rozemuller A, Van Gool WA, Hoozemans J. The significance of neuroinflammation in understanding Alzheimer's disease. Journal of Neural Transmission. 2006;**113**:1685-1695

[161] Hensley K, Mhatre M, Mou S, Pye QN, Stewart C, West M, et al. On the relation of oxidative stress to neuroinflammation: Lessons learned from the G93A-SOD1 mouse model of amyotrophic lateral sclerosis. Antioxidants & Redox Signaling. 2006;**8**:2075-2087

[162] Minghetti L. Role of inflammation in neurodegenerative diseases. Current Opinion in Neurology. 2005;**18**:315-321

[163] Taupin P. Adult neurogenesis, neuroinflammation and therapeutic potential of adult neural stem cells. International Journal of Medical Sciences. 2008;**5**:127

[164] Posey KA, Clegg DJ, Printz RL, Byun J, Morton GJ, Vivekanandan-Giri A, et al. Hypothalamic proinflammatory lipid accumulation, inflammation, and insulin resistance in rats fed a high-fat diet. American Journal of Physiology-Endocrinology and Metabolism. 2009;**296**:E1003-E1012

[165] Kleinridders A, Schenten D, Könner AC, Belgardt BF, Mauer J, Okamura T, et al. MyD88 signaling in the CNS is required for development of fatty acid-induced leptin resistance and diet-induced obesity. Cell Metabolism. 2009;**10**:249-259

[166] Meng Q, Cai D. Defective hypothalamic autophagy directs the central pathogenesis of obesity via the IκB kinase β (IKKβ)/NF-κB pathway. Journal of Biological Chemistry. 2011;**286**:32324-32332

[167] Milanski M, Degasperi G, Coope A, Morari J, Denis R, Cintra DE, et al. Saturated fatty acids produce an inflammatory response predominantly through the activation of TLR4 signaling in hypothalamus: Implications for the pathogenesis of obesity. Journal of Neuroscience. 2009;**29**:359-370

[168] Oh IS, Thaler JP, Ogimoto K, Wisse BE, Morton GJ, Schwartz MW. Central administration of interleukin-4 exacerbates hypothalamic inflammation and weight gain during high-fat feeding. American Journal of Physiology-Endocrinology and Metabolism. 2010;**299**:E47-E53

[169] Purkayastha S, Zhang H, Zhang G, Ahmed Z, Wang Y, Cai D. Neural dysregulation of peripheral insulin action and blood pressure by brain endoplasmic reticulum stress. Proceedings of the National Academy of Sciences. 2011;**108**:2939-2944

[170] Ballard C, Gauthier S, Corbett A, Brayne C, Aarsland D, Jones E. Alzheimer's disease. The Lancet. 2011;**377**:1019-1031

[171] Beydoun MA, Beydoun H, Wang Y. Obesity and central obesity as risk factors for incident dementia and its subtypes: A systematic review and meta-analysis. Obesity Reviews. 2008;**9**:204-218

[172] Hamer M, Chida Y. Physical activity and risk of neurodegenerative disease: A systematic review of prospective evidence. Psychological Medicine. 2009;**39**:3-11

[173] Lu F-P, Lin K-P, Kuo H-K. Diabetes and the risk of multi-system aging phenotypes: A systematic review and meta-analysis. PLoS One. 2009;**4**:e4144

[174] Grote HE, Hannan AJ. Regulators of adult neurogenesis in the healthy and diseased brain. Clinical and Experimental Pharmacology and Physiology. 2007;**34**:533-545

[175] Monje ML, Toda H, Palmer TD. Inflammatory blockade restores adult hippocampal neurogenesis. Science. 2003;**302**:1760-1765

[176] Lee DA, Bedont JL, Pak T, Wang H, Song J, Miranda-Angulo A, et al. Tanycytes of the hypothalamic median eminence form a diet-responsive neurogenic niche. Nature Neuroscience. 2012;**15**:700-702

[177] Mcnay DE, Briançon N, Kokoeva MV, Maratos-Flier E, Flier JS. Remodeling of the arcuate nucleus energy-balance circuit is inhibited in obese mice. The Journal of Clinical Investigation. 2012;**122**:142-152

[178] Drapeau E, Montaron M-F, Aguerre S, Abrous DN. Learning-induced survival of new neurons depends on the cognitive status of aged rats. Journal of Neuroscience. 2007;**27**:6037-6044

[179] Gould E, Beylin A, Tanapat P, Reeves A, Shors TJ. Learning enhances adult neurogenesis in the hippocampal formation. Nature Neuroscience. 1999a;**2**:260-265

[180] Shors TJ, Miesegaes G, Beylin A, Zhao M, Rydel T, Gould E. Neurogenesis in the adult is involved in the formation of trace memories. Nature. 2001;**410**:372-376

[181] Leal G, Bramham C, Duarte C. BDNF and hippocampal synaptic plasticity. Vitamins and Hormones. 2017;**104**:153-195

[182] Reichelt AC, Hare DJ, Bussey TJ, Saksida LM. Perineuronal nets: Plasticity, protection, and therapeutic potential. Trends in Neurosciences. 2019;**42**:458-470

[183] Cui Y, Cao K, Lin H, Cui S, Shen C, Wen W, et al. Early-life stress induces depression-like behavior and synaptic-plasticity changes in a maternal separation rat model: Gender difference and metabolomics study. Frontiers in Pharmacology. 2020;**11**:102

[184] Jackson J, Jambrina E, Li J, Marston H, Menzies F, Phillips K, et al. Targeting the synapse in Alzheimer's disease. Frontiers in Neuroscience. 2019;**13**:735

[185] Ramiro-Cortés Y, Hobbiss AF, Israely I. Synaptic competition in structural plasticity and cognitive function. Philosophical Transactions of the Royal Society B: Biological Sciences. 2014;**369**:20130157

[186] Abidin İ, Aydin-Abidin S, Bodur A, Ince İ, Alver A. Brain-derived neurotropic factor (BDNF) heterozygous mice are more susceptible to synaptic protein loss in cerebral cortex during high fat diet. Archives of Physiology and Biochemistry. 2018;**124**:442-447

[187] Arnold SE, Lucki I, Brookshire BR, Carlson GC, Browne CA, Kazi H, et al. High fat diet produces brain insulin resistance, synaptodendritic abnormalities and altered behavior

in mice. Neurobiology of Disease. 2014;**67**:79-87

[188] Bhat NR, Thirumangalakudi L. Increased tau phosphorylation and impaired brain insulin/IGF signaling in mice fed a high fat/high cholesterol diet. Journal of Alzheimer's Disease. 2013;**36**:781-789

[189] Bocarsly ME, Fasolino M, Kane GA, Lamarca EA, Kirschen GW, Karatsoreos IN, et al. Obesity diminishes synaptic markers, alters microglial morphology, and impairs cognitive function. Proceedings of the National Academy of Sciences. 2015;**112**:15731-15736

[190] Cavaliere G, Viggiano E, Trinchese G, De Filippo C, Messina A, Monda V, et al. Long feeding high-fat diet induces hypothalamic oxidative stress and inflammation, and prolonged hypothalamic AMPK activation in rat animal model. Frontiers in Physiology. 2018;**9**:818

[191] Hao S, Dey A, Yu X, Stranahan AM. Dietary obesity reversibly induces synaptic stripping by microglia and impairs hippocampal plasticity. Brain, Behavior, and Immunity. 2016;**51**:230-239

[192] Papazoglou IK, Jean A, Gertler A, Taouis M, Vacher C-M. Hippocampal GSK3β as a molecular link between obesity and depression. Molecular Neurobiology. 2015;**52**:363-374

[193] Puig KL, Floden AM, Adhikari R, Golovko MY, Combs CK. Amyloid precursor protein and proinflammatory changes are regulated in brain and adipose tissue in a murine model of high fat diet-induced obesity. PLoS One. 2012;**7**:e30378

[194] Valcarcel-Ares MN, Tucsek Z, Kiss T, Giles CB, Tarantini S, Yabluchanskiy A, et al. Obesity in aging exacerbates neuroinflammation, dysregulating synaptic function-related genes and altering eicosanoid synthesis in the mouse hippocampus: Potential role in impaired synaptic plasticity and cognitive decline. The Journals of Gerontology: Series A. 2019;**74**:290-298

[195] Dutheil S, Ota KT, Wohleb ES, Rasmussen K, Duman RS. High-fat diet induced anxiety and anhedonia: Impact on brain homeostasis and inflammation. Neuropsychopharmacology. 2016;**41**:1874-1887

[196] Salameh TS, Mortell WG, Logsdon AF, Butterfield DA, Banks WA. Disruption of the hippocampal and hypothalamic blood–brain barrier in a diet-induced obese model of type II diabetes: Prevention and treatment by the mitochondrial carbonic anhydrase inhibitor, topiramate. Fluids and Barriers of the CNS. 2019;**16**:1-17

[197] Tongiorgi E. Activity-dependent expression of brain-derived neurotrophic factor in dendrites: Facts and open questions. Neuroscience Research. 2008;**61**:335-346

[198] Sharma S, Fulton S. Diet-induced obesity promotes depressive-like behaviour that is associated with neural adaptations in brain reward circuitry. International Journal of Obesity. 2013;**37**:382-389

[199] Notaras M, van den Buuse M. Brain-derived neurotrophic factor (BDNF): Novel insights into regulation and genetic variation. The Neuroscientist. 2019;**25**:434-454

[200] Vanevski F, Xu B. Molecular and neural bases underlying roles of BDNF in the control of body weight. Frontiers in Neuroscience. 2013;**7**:37

[201] Gupta S, Mishra R, Kusum S, Spedding M, Meiri K, Gressens P, et al. GAP-43 is essential for the neurotrophic effects of BDNF and positive AMPA receptor modulator S18986. Cell Death & Differentiation. 2009;**16**:624-637

[202] Wang Z, Ge Q, Wu Y, Zhang J, Gu Q, Han J. Impairment of long-term memory by a short-term high-fat diet via hippocampal oxidative stress and alterations in synaptic plasticity. Neuroscience. 2020;**424**:24-33

[203] Wu A, Ying Z, Gomez-Pinilla F. The interplay between oxidative stress and brain-derived neurotrophic factor modulates the outcome of a saturated fat diet on synaptic plasticity and cognition. European Journal of Neuroscience. 2004;**19**:1699-1707

[204] Jovanovic J, Czernik AJ, Fienberg AA, Greengard P, Sihra TS. Synapsins as mediators of BDNF-enhanced neurotransmitter release. Nature Neuroscience. 2000;**3**:323-329

[205] Pandit M, Behl T, Sachdeva M, Arora S. Role of brain derived neurotropic factor in obesity. Obesity Medicine. 2020;**17**:100189

[206] Criscuolo C, Fabiani C, Bonadonna C, Origlia N, Domenici L. BDNF prevents amyloid-dependent impairment of LTP in the entorhinal cortex by attenuating p38 MAPK phosphorylation. Neurobiology of Aging. 2015;**36**:1303-1309

[207] Kurhe Y, Mahesh R, Devadoss T. Novel 5-HT3 receptor antagonist QCM-4 attenuates depressive-like phenotype associated with obesity in high-fat-diet-fed mice. Psychopharmacology. 2017;**234**:1165-1179

[208] Park HR, Park M, Choi J, Park K-Y, Chung HY, Lee J. A high-fat diet impairs neurogenesis: Involvement of lipid peroxidation and brain-derived neurotrophic factor. Neuroscience Letters. 2010;**482**:235-239

[209] Reichelt AC, Maniam J, Westbrook RF, Morris MJ. Dietary-induced obesity disrupts trace fear conditioning and decreases hippocampal reelin expression. Brain, Behavior, and Immunity. 2015;**43**:68-75

[210] Jin Y, Sun LH, Yang W, Cui RJ, Xu SB. The role of BDNF in the neuroimmune axis regulation of mood disorders. Frontiers in Neurology. 2019;**10**:515

[211] Puig KL, Brose SA, Zhou X, Sens MA, Combs GF, Jensen MD, et al. Amyloid precursor protein modulates macrophage phenotype and diet-dependent weight gain. Scientific Reports. 2017;**7**:1-14

[212] Mehta P, Pirttila T, Patrick B, Barshatzky M, Mehta S. Amyloid β protein 1-40 and 1-42 levels in matched cerebrospinal fluid and plasma from patients with Alzheimer disease. Neuroscience Letters. 2001;**304**:102-106

[213] Ismail N, Ismail M, Azmi NH, Bakar MFA, Yida Z, Abdullah MA, et al. Thymoquinone-rich fraction nanoemulsion (TQRFNE) decreases Aβ40 and Aβ42 levels by modulating APP processing, up-regulating IDE and LRP1, and down-regulating BACE1 and RAGE in response to high fat/cholesterol diet-induced rats. Biomedicine & Pharmacotherapy. 2017;**95**:780-788

[214] Nuzzo D, Baldassano S, Amato A, Picone P, Galizzi G, Caldara GF, et al. Glucagon-like peptide-2 reduces the obesity-associated inflammation in the brain. Neurobiology of Disease. 2019;**121**:296-304

[215] Lee YH, Tharp WG, Maple RL, Nair S, Permana PA, Pratley RE. Amyloid precursor protein expression is upregulated in adipocytes in obesity. Obesity. 2008;**16**:1493-1500

[216] Sommer G, Kralisch S, Lipfert J, Weise S, Krause K, Jessnitzer B, et al. Amyloid precursor protein expression is induced by tumor necrosis factor α in 3T3-L1 adipocytes. Journal of Cellular Biochemistry. 2009;**108**:1418-1422

[217] Tarantini S, Valcarcel-Ares MN, Yabluchanskiy A, Tucsek Z, Hertelendy P, Kiss T, et al. Nrf2 deficiency exacerbates obesity-induced oxidative stress, neurovascular dysfunction, blood–brain barrier disruption, neuroinflammation, amyloidogenic gene expression, and cognitive decline in mice, mimicking the aging phenotype. The Journals of Gerontology: Series A. 2018;**73**:853-863

[218] Kohjima M, Sun Y, Chan L. Increased food intake leads to obesity and insulin resistance in the tg2576 Alzheimer's disease mouse model. Endocrinology. 2010;**151**:1532-1540

[219] Thirumangalakudi L, Prakasam A, Zhang R, Bimonte-Nelson H, Sambamurti K, Kindy MS, et al. High cholesterol-induced neuroinflammation and amyloid precursor protein processing correlate with loss of working memory in mice. Journal of Neurochemistry. 2008;**106**:475-485

[220] Nakandakari SCBR, Munoz VR, Kuga GK, Gaspar RC, Sant'ana MR, Pavan ICB, et al. Short-term high-fat diet modulates several inflammatory, ER stress, and apoptosis markers in the hippocampus of young mice. Brain, Behavior, and Immunity. 2019;**79**:284-293

[221] Frühbeis C, Fröhlich D, Kuo WP, Krämer-Albers E-M. Extracellular vesicles as mediators of neuron-glia communication. Frontiers in Cellular Neuroscience. 2013;**7**:182

[222] Duffy C, Hofmeister J, Nixon JP, Butterick T. High fat diet increases cognitive decline and neuroinflammation in a model of orexin loss. Neurobiology of Learning and Memory. 2019;**157**:41-47

[223] Vinuesa A, Bentivegna M, Calfa G, Filipello F, Pomilio C, Bonaventura MM, et al. Early exposure to a high-fat diet impacts on hippocampal plasticity: Implication of microglia-derived exosome-like extracellular vesicles. Molecular Neurobiology. 2019;**56**:5075-5094

[224] Cope EC, Lamarca EA, Monari PK, Olson LB, Martinez S, Zych AD, et al. Microglia play an active role in obesity-associated cognitive decline. Journal of Neuroscience. 2018;**38**:8889-8904

[225] Battú CE, Rieger D, Loureiro S, Furtado GV, Bock H, Saraiva-Pereira M-L, et al. Alterations of PI3K and Akt signaling pathways in the hippocampus and hypothalamus of Wistar rats treated with highly palatable food. Nutritional Neuroscience. 2012;**15**:10-17

[226] Kothari V, Luo Y, Tornabene T, O'Neill AM, Greene MW, Geetha T, et al. High fat diet induces brain insulin resistance and cognitive impairment in mice. Biochimica et Biophysica Acta (BBA)-Molecular Basis of Disease. 2017;**1863**:499-508

[227] Wijtenburg SA, Kapogiannis D, Korenic SA, Mullins RJ, Tran J, Gaston FE, et al. Brain insulin resistance and altered brain glucose are related to memory impairments in

schizophrenia. Schizophrenia Research. 2019;**208**:324-330

[228] Matsuzaki T, Sasaki K, Tanizaki Y, Hata J, Fujimi K, Matsui Y, et al. Insulin resistance is associated with the pathology of Alzheimer disease: The Hisayama study. Neurology. 2010;**75**:764-770

[229] Lomniczi A, Ojeda SR. A role for glial cells of the neuroendocrine brain in the central control of female sexual development. In: Astrocytes in (Patho) Physiology of the Nervous System. Springer; 2009

[230] Boeckers TM, Bockmann J, Kreutz MR, Gundelfinger ED. ProSAP/shank proteins–a family of higher order organizing molecules of the postsynaptic density with an emerging role in human neurological disease. Journal of Neurochemistry. 2002;**81**:903-910

[231] Mielke JG, Nicolitch K, Avellaneda V, Earlam K, Ahuja T, Mealing G, et al. Longitudinal study of the effects of a high-fat diet on glucose regulation, hippocampal function, and cerebral insulin sensitivity in C57BL/6 mice. Behavioural Brain Research. 2006;**175**:374-382

[232] Vander Heide LP, Kamal A, Artola A, Gispen WH, Ramakers GM. Insulin modulates hippocampal activity-dependent synaptic plasticity in a N-methyl-d-aspartate receptor and phosphatidyl-inositol-3-kinase-dependent manner. Journal of Neurochemistry. 2005;**94**:1158-1166

[233] Anfal A-D, Ahram M, Hayder A. Effects of obesity on hippocampus function: Synaptic plasticity hypothesis. Obesity Medicine. 2020;**19**:100246

[234] Dingess PM, Darling RA, Kurt Dolence E, Culver BW, Brown TE. Exposure to a diet high in fat attenuates dendritic spine density in the medial prefrontal cortex. Brain Structure and Function. 2017;**222**:1077-1085

[235] Uranga RM, Bruce-Keller AJ, Morrison CD, Fernandez-Kim SO, Ebenezer PJ, Zhang L, et al. Intersection between metabolic dysfunction, high fat diet consumption, and brain aging. Journal of Neurochemistry. 2010;**114**:344-361

[236] Magariños AM, Mcewen BS. Experimental diabetes in rats causes hippocampal dendritic and synaptic reorganization and increased glucocorticoid reactivity to stress. Proceedings of the National Academy of Sciences. 2000;**97**:11056-11061

[237] Pamidi N, Satheesha Nayak BN. Effect of streptozotocin induced diabetes on rat hippocampus. Bratislavské Lekárske Listy. 2012;**113**:583-588

[238] Ramos-Rodriguez JJ, Molina-Gil S, Ortiz-Barajas O, Jimenez-Palomares M, Perdomo G, Cozar-Castellano I, et al. Central proliferation and neurogenesis is impaired in type 2 diabetes and prediabetes animal models. PLoS One. 2014;**9**:e89229

[239] Stranahan AM, Norman ED, Lee K, Cutler RG, Telljohann RS, Egan JM, et al. Diet-induced insulin resistance impairs hippocampal synaptic plasticity and cognition in middle-aged rats. Hippocampus. 2008;**18**:1085-1088

[240] Karimi SA, Salehi I, Komaki A, Sarihi A, Zarei M, Shahidi S. Effect of high-fat diet and antioxidants on hippocampal long-term potentiation in rats: An in vivo study. Brain Research. 2013;**1539**:1-6

[241] Yoon G, Cho KA, Song J, Kim Y-K. Transcriptomic analysis of high fat diet

fed mouse brain cortex. Frontiers in Genetics. 2019;**10**:83

[242] Lindqvist A, Mohapel P, Bouter B, Frielingsdorf H, Pizzo D, Brundin P, et al. High-fat diet impairs hippocampal neurogenesis in male rats. European Journal of Neurology. 2006;**13**:1385-1388

Chapter 5

Obesity: A Prerequisite for Major Chronic Illnesses

Hafeez Abiola Afolabi, Zaidi Zakaria, Salzihan Md. Salleh, Ewe Seng Ch'ng, Siti Norasikin Mohd Nafi, Ahmad Aizat Bin Abdul Aziz, Sameer Badri Al-Mhanna, Ahmad Adebayo Irekeola, Yusuf Wada and Abubakar Bishir Daku

Abstract

Obesity is rampantly soaring at an alarming rate globally and simultaneously causing an increased incidence, and predisposition to various comorbidities. obesity is body mass index of >30kg/m^2, while <18kg/m^2 is underweight. The world at large fails to recognize obesity as an inevitable disease that requires strict measures to control this modifiable risk factor. W.H.O news release reported that over one billion people globally are obese among which 650 million were adults, 340 million were adolescents, and 39 million were children. The lowest obesity prevalence was reported in Timor Leste at 3.80%, Bangladesh at 3.60%, and Vietnam at 2.10% while the highest were noted in Nauru at 61%, cook island at 55.9%, and Palau at 55.3%. obesity is the most prevailing health problem (15% globally) associated with an increased propensity for development of several medical illnesses, obesity-associated adverse outcomes causing fatal complications that are difficult to manage, and premature mortality. The obese often feel they are not socially cared for by society and are accorded limited time by physicians who don't view their health concerns from their own perspectives. Thus, making them pessimistic from low self-esteem and discrimination, body shaming, and stigmatization. They eventually develop depressive-anxiety disorder because of distrust insight.

Keywords: obesity, overweight, body mass index (BMI), comorbid, chronic diseases, obesity prevalence

1. Introduction

Obesity is exponentially rising at an alarming rate and simultaneously causing an increased incidence of substantial adverse effects, and predisposition to various comorbidities such as osteoarthritis, coronary heart disease, and hypertension [1, 2]. Globally, obesity has precipitously grown to become a pandemic in all countries due to several contributing factors from vicissitudes in human lifestyles and societal norms, in addition to the multi-factorial existing causes of obesity: genetics, dietary intake, and lifestyle modification [3–5]. Putting all these puzzles together, obesity represents a major healthcare crisis, both medically and economically around the globe [6–8].

Identifying and categorizing obese from the non-obese or even from the overweight that is deemed borderline between the non-obese and the obese individuals involve the classification based on Body Mass Index (BMI). Obesity classifications and definitions vary but, by and large, the definition by the World Health Organization (WHO) is commonly employed as the gold standard. It defined obesity as a Body Mass Index (BMI) of 30 kg/m^2 or more, 25–29.9 kg/m^2 as overweight, and 18.5–24.5 kg/m^2 as normal BMI while less than 18 are considered underweight [9].

2. Global epidemiology of obesity

On March 4, 2022, the news release theme by the WHO [10] on "World Obesity Day 2022" was "Accelerating action to stop obesity" but will it ever come about? Well, the answer is feasible! Less likely of course because the world has yet to recognize obesity as a disease or pandemic that is inevitable if strict measures are not taken to control the modifiable risk factors that are most probable factors. As such the WHO is encouraging countries to act more to overturn this foreseeable and escapable health crisis. According to the WHO news release, greater than 1 billion people globally are obese of which 650 million were adults, 340 million were adolescents, and 39 million were children [11]. More astonishing is the fact that this number is still increasing. WHO estimates that by 2025, about 167 million people: adults and children will become less healthy because of being overweight or obese [12]. Between 2011 and 2014, the gross proportion of the prevalence of obesity among adults in the United States was 36.5%, by 2016, the figure rises more, 38.9% of US adults were obese while 7.6% were classified as severely obese [13, 14]. Between 2017 and 2018, 41.9% of women 20 years and more of the US were said to be obese [15]. In 2016, 13% of adult globally were said to be obese [16]. Overall, middle-aged individuals 40–59 years old (40.2%) and older aged individuals 60 and above (37.0%) had a greater incidence of obesity than younger adults aged 20–39 (32.3%) [17]. Overall gender predilection shows that women (38.3%) had a greater propensity for obesity than men (34.3%) [18].

Heightened prevalence of obesity and overweight are being reported in several nooks and crannies of the globe: in the Middle East region, the prevalence of obesity and overweight among people 40 years old and above between 2000 and 2006 was 21.17% but increased to 33.4% between 2014 and 2020 [19]. In Europe, obesity prevalence is estimated at 60% among adults populations [20], approximately even higher than 60% in Asia [2]. According to the [21], over half of the British population were said to be overweight between 1980 and 1995, the prevalence of obesity in Britain also doubled from 8% to 15% in 2016, in fact it was projected that by 2050, 15% and 62% of females in social class I and class V will be obese [22]. Most of South America and parts of Asia reported it at 16.4% from 2015 to 2019 in China [23]. Country-wise according to the world population review, the highest obesity prevalence was recorded in countries such as Nauru 61%, Cook Island 55.9%, Palau 55.3%, Kuwait 37.9%. In the US, obesity prevalence has risen from 19.4% in 1997 to 31.4% in 2017 [24] and 36.20% in 2022 while the least was reported in Japan 4.30%, India 3.90%, Timor Leste 3.80%, Bangladesh 3.60%, and Vietnam 2.10% (full description in **Figure 1**).

Globally, the proportion of obesity is higher in women than in men by approximately 1.6-fold, at least to a certain extent, that a female higher occurrence rate would be anticipated, owing to the biologically higher ratio of body fat in women [25].

In some societies, the rate of obesity is higher in lower socio-economic classes, this can be attributed to the greater degree of fast-food restaurants in low-income districts, the higher price of healthful diets, safety fears that inhibit walking and other outdoor activities, and greater economic woes [26–28].

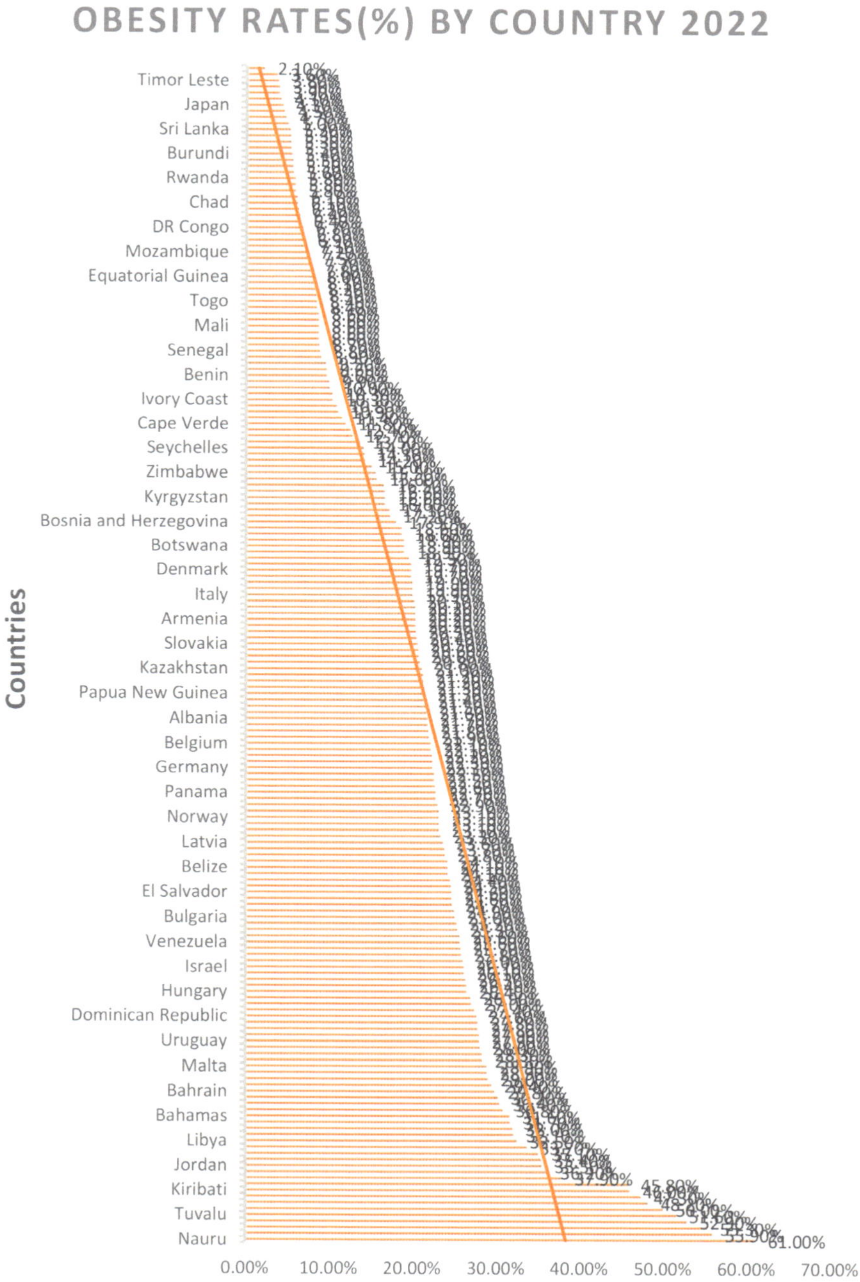

Figure 1.
Illustration of obesity prevalence by countries. (Obesity Rates by Country 2022: https://worldpopulationreview.com/country-rankings/obesity-rates-by-country).

3. Etiology of obesity

Not only does obesity affects 15% of the global populace, but it is also an underlying cause for several other chronic diseases, yet, surprisingly, it has until recently been regarded as a disease. The genesis of obesity is multi-factorial likewise the epidemic is almost certainly associated with rising sedentary daily life combined with increased desire for satiety satisfaction. However, this is not always so for every obese individual because there is substantial evidence of genetics: obesity-inherited link in the vast majority of traits.

Obesity in the form of weight gain is a continuous process resulting from the constellation of genetic, behavioral, environmental, physiological, social, and cultural factors that ultimately lead to energy imbalance and accumulation of excessive fat deposits [29, 30]. A heightened desire for taste satisfaction and abundant inexpensive, energy-dense readily available fast food increases energy consumption, because these promote feasting out of home, provides varieties of food options and large portions [31]. These eventually will lead to an imbalance between energy intake and energy output. The identification and understanding of the neuronal substrates mediating overeating (after consumption of a high-energy meal) explain the increased neural activity in the amygdala: the interstitial nucleus of the posterior limb of the anterior commissure (IPAC). The neurons in the IPAC system can be activated and switched on after eating or upon food smelling which eventually increases satiety in eating habits [32]. Being a complex system, the amygdala interface with other limbic structures to regulate emotion, learning, and behavior, through these interactions, it modulates and plays a role in the emotional-eating pattern that eventually promotes the overeating response [33, 34]. However, there are other mechanisms for increasing weight gain and many other mechanisms are still unclear.

Leptin, a neuromodulator protein formed predominantly in the white subcutaneous adipose tissue is a crucial body-weight regulator in the human feeding and satiety cycle [35, 36]. Leptin sends satiety impulses to the hypothalamus and thus decreasing food intake and fat storage while ensuring modulation of energy expenditure and carbohydrate metabolism, and finally averting excessive weight gain [37]. Most of the people living with obesity are not leptin-deficient but, they actually have a leptin-resistant condition. Thence, they have higher levels of circulating leptin. Women have higher leptin levels than their male counterparts, and these higher leptin levels have a direct relationship with potentially higher BMI in females.

Among other pathways are Hypertrophic-hypercellular obesity wherein the adipose tissues or fat cells increases in size and number and are manifested as abdominal obesity, commonly noticeable in adulthood [38, 39]. With some of these primary adipocytes-secreting pro-inflammatory products: Tumor necrosis factor–alpha TNF-α, Interleukin 6 IL-6, Monocyte chemoattractant protein–1 (MCP-1), etc. acting as active metabolites that support lipid storage, fatty acid synthesis and lipids exudate from adipocytes deposits [40, 41]. Effect of hormones, neurotransmitters, and neurogenic signals on feeding habits are also worth mentioning. Certain hormones such as endocannabinoids increases appetite, promote nutrient uptake, and promote lipogenesis. There are other varieties of gut hormones such as glucagon-like peptide-1 (GLP-1), neuropeptide YY (PYY), and cholecystokinin that act substantially to induce satiety to affect eating habits [42, 43].

The benefit here is that understanding these pathways also gives science possible therapeutic targets for obesity control. Ultimately, the occurrence or increase of obesity resides in an imbalance between energy intake and energy expenditure over a lengthy period, therefore the etiology can be seen as surplus energy intake relative to daily energy expenditure, or as low energy expenditure relative to daily energy intake.

4. Obesity and other chronic disease pathophysiology

Obesity-related health conditions are numerous and associated with increased morbidity and greater mortality. The major obesity-related comorbidities include cardiovascular disease (majorly heart disease and stroke), type 2 diabetes, dyslipidemia, musculoskeletal disorders (osteoarthritis especially), and certain cancers (endometrial, breast, and colon) [44]. These illnesses are underlying causes for premature death and substantial health disability. Expert reviews by Chetambath et al. [45] indicated that a BMI of 25–28.9 kg/m^2 is associated with a relative risk of 1.72 for coronary heart disease the risk gradually rises with an increasing BMI; for BMIs more than 33 kg/m^2, the relative risk is 3.44. A similar trend was also reported between obesity and stroke respectively [45]. In general, obesity is reported to increase mortality rate from cardiovascular disease by 4-fold and by 2-fold for cancer-related death. Moreso severely obese (BMI $\geq$40) showed a 6–12-fold probability of an all-cause mortality rate, a reduced life expectancy by 20 years in men, and approximately 5 years in women [46–48]. Although there is no definitive or no cause-and-effect association that undoubtedly established obesity direct cause of these comorbidities, however, improvement of these illnesses after significant weight reduction indicates that high body mass index plays an important role in the propagation of the diseases [49, 50]. A schematic diagram is illustrated in **Figure 2**.

Hypertension (high blood pressure) is among the foremost prevalent comorbidity associated with obesity, and in turn is a crucial risk factor for stroke, myocardial infarction, heart failure, and chronic renal disease [51, 52]. Independent risk factors such as high body mass index and/or overweight are 65–75% linked to primary (essential) hypertension [53], with at least 72% contribution in hypertension and/or T2DM

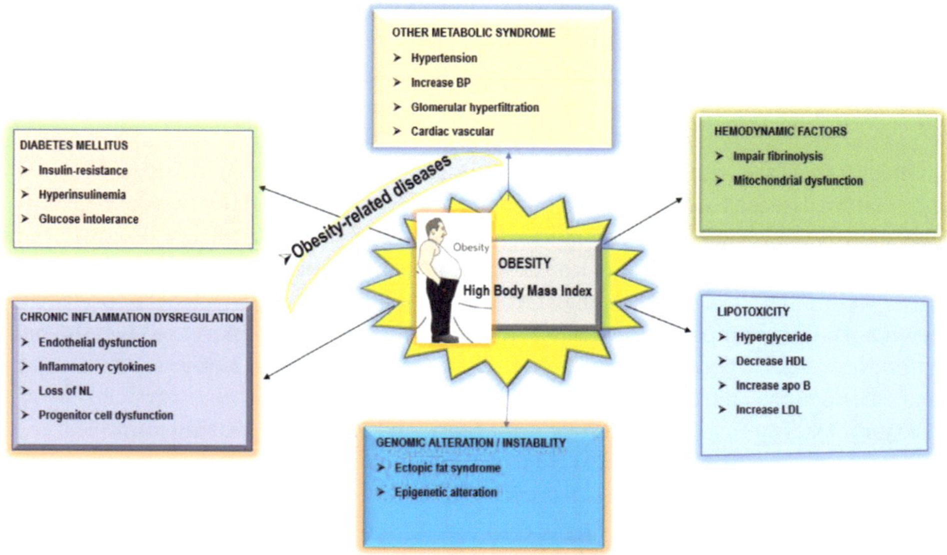

Figure 2.
Schematic diagram of obesity-related chronic disease.

diagnosed patients with end-stage renal disease, although the mechanism is yet to be fully understood [53]. Nonetheless, significant progress has been made in explaining some of the intricate relationships between renal, hormonal, and neurological system components that connect excessive adiposity with high blood pressure. Literally, the amount of blood flowing through the body increases with increased body weight, and this place additional pressure on artery walls, leading to increased arterial blood pressure (hypertension). Besides this, being overweight also increases the heart rate and thus makes blood flow within the blood vessel harder. Obesity generally reduces the parasympathetic pitch and intensifies sympathetic activity. These autonomic activity modifications cause increased heart rate, decreases heart rate variability, and reduced baroreflex sensitivity. According to the Nurses' Health Study in the United State, women who had a BMI above 32 had a four times higher mortality rate from cardiovascular disease than those who had a BMI under 19 [54–56].

Pulmonary function is also a prognosticator of various recurring illnesses even though various research outcomes on the obesity-lung function association are inconsistent. Nonetheless, a lot of research have reported central obesity as a reliable indicator of poor lung function [57]. Obesity is a serious mitigating condition that is frequently associated with respiratory problems, thus reducing the exercise-tolerance capacity of the obese perhaps due to early exhaustion. Obesity is the main culprit in obstructive sleep apnea, a condition that disrupts sleep, produces snoring and apneic episodes, and lowers oxygen saturation to levels associated with potentially fatal cardiac rhythms [58]. Due to modifications in respiratory mechanism and bronchospasm produced by gastroesophageal reflux illness, obesity makes respiratory symptoms such as dyspnea worse [59]. Obesity-lung function association by most studies has focused on the association between lung function and central obesity and central obesity indicators, however, the relationship is inversely purported while for some, the association is weak and for others, there is an independent obesity indicators-lung function interaction [59, 60]. Obesity especially central obesity restricts lung compliance function due to diaphragm-reduced movement (expansion-relaxation function) which eventually limits the respiratory functional capacity of the lungs leading to decreased lung function i.e. FVC and FEV1 in people with central obesity than when compared to the normal population [23]. An alternative possible mechanism is a reduction in the functional pulmonary capacity due to increased deposition of adipose tissues in the pulmonary compartment and respiratory-supporting tissues such as in the abdomen and surrounding viscera [61].

Obesity increases the risk of arthritis especially primary osteoarthritis (OA), a degenerative disease that causes excessive matrix degradation on the weight-bearing joints such as the hips, knees, and ankles as well as the possibility of foot discomfort and plantar fasciitis, all of which may lead to secondary limitations in physical activity and further weight gain [62]. Although osteoarthritis etiology is multi-factorial, obesity is labeled as the single most predisposing modifiable factor to OA. Increased weight-bearing condition such as obesity causes changes in the articular joint bony structures (joint space narrowing). There is subchondral ablation of the articular bony-cartilage layer of the joint leading to a greater loss of joint space on the weight-bearing joint [63], the proteoglycans level drops significantly to a critical level that makes the articular cartilage to become soften and lose its elasticity character, thus, further compromising joint surface integrity [64]. The resulting features of osteoarthritis arise i.e., pain, stiffness, and reduced movement because of the inconvenience caused by overloading (obesity). Significant weight loss is linked to a decrease in arthritic joint discomfort, and in some people, it may prevent or delay the need for joint replacement surgery [65].

Obesity has been reported to have a direct correlation with non-alcoholic fatty liver disease, increased gastric disease and hepatobiliary diseases are also associated with obesity [66]. Because of their increased biliary excretion of cholesterol, obese people are more likely to develop gallstones, cholecystitis, and biliary dyskinesia (biliary colic without cholelithiasis) [67]. Although cholesterol is eliminated and released when lowering fat storage, it may solidify in the gallbladder and raise the risk of cholelithiasis and cholecystitis. Small quantities of fat consumed every day as part of a weight reduction plan may empty the gallbladder and lower this risk. Non-alcoholic fatty liver disease caused by obesity may lead to cirrhosis and liver failure but is often preventable or mitigated by weight loss [68].

There is a strong evidence indicating that obesity is directly associated with cancer, there are prevalence evidence of obesity propensity for certain types of cancer: endometrial cancer is 7-fold and 2–4 times increased in the severely obese and obese/overweight respectively, esophageal adenocarcinoma is about 4–8 fold high in severely obese and 2.4–2.7 times more likely among obese individuals [69, 70], gastric cancer, kidney cancer and liver cancer are 2-fold higher with obesity, for others, its 1.5 fold likely for colorectal cancer,1.6-fold for gallbladder cancer, 1.2–1.4 and 0.8 times for breast postmenopausal and premenopausal cancer respectively, 1.1 times for ovarian cancer, and 1.3 times for liver cancer [69, 70].

Obesity and cancer remain a topic of investigation. Being overweight or obese can induce alterations in the body tissues that increases cancer propensity [71]. These alterations comprise long- *there are prevalence evidence of obesity propensity* levels of other hormones, such as insulin, insulin-like growth factor, sex hormones, as well as alteration of adipocytokine levels like leptins, adiponectin, and visfatin [72]. How obesity increase risk of cancer involves several possible mechanisms including: (1) Fat tissue-increase of estrogen and thus heightened risk of cancer of the breast, ovaries, endometrial etc., (2) hyperinsulinemia from elevated free fatty acid levels in the obese that cause insulin resistance and the eventual increased blood glucose that increases the risk hyperinsulinemia, (3) low-grade inflammation and oxidative stress that affect growth-promoting cytokines and immune modulation, and (4) intestinal flora microbiomes alteration [73].

Very astonishing to know that 20% of all cancer cases are thought to be associated with excess weight gain, and obesity [74], although tumors' etiologic routes are driven by several factors and the mechanisms varies with respect to tumor-type. People living with obesity have an approximately 1.5–3.5-fold greater chance of developing certain cancer-types compared with normal-weight people [75], however, this latter statement does not imply that an overweight or obese person will definitely develop cancer, but the chances rise. Being overweight or obese raises the risk of 13 cancer-types namely: cancer of breast in post-menopausal, ovarian, esophageal, thyroid, pancreas, kidney, hepatocyte, stomach, gallbladder, myeloma, and meningioma of the brain [76]. In Europe, more than 1 in 20 cancer incidents are attributed to excessive weight in the UK [77]. Breast cancer risk is lower among those who lose weight, especially postmenopausal women. Less robust data exist for cancer patients, but observations pointing to a long history of poor outcomes for obese women with breast cancer are well detailed [76]. Even though there are different ideas about how obesity affects the outcome of different cancers, there is much evidence that exercise is advantageous for breast and colon cancer [78, 79]. According to a meta-analysis research that was published in 2002, obesity was the root cause of 11% of instances of colon cancer, 9% of cases of postmenopausal breast cancer, 39% of cases of endometrial cancer, 25% of cases of kidney cancer, and 37% of cases of esophageal cancer [80].

Although there are few studies that look at weight or changes in weight with survival after cancer diagnosis but obesity and poor outcomes for breast cancer survivors have long been reported by researchers. The majority of evidence indicates that being overweight/obese at diagnosis is the main lifestyle risk factor for having a poor prognosis for breast cancer and a poor quality of life status [81] thus, supporting the growing evidence demonstrating that gaining weight after diagnosis increases risk [82]. The importance of energy balance after breast cancer is further supported by research showing that physical activity reduces the risk of breast cancer recurrence [83] as intervention trials of diet and exercise showed longer disease-free survival among intervention groups of which lost significant weight than the control group [84].

On the other hand obesity is one of the most significant risk factors for developing stroke [85]. Both genders and several ethnic communities, including Caucasians, Chinese, and Japanese people, have shown a substantial connection between obesity and an elevated risk for ischemic stroke [86]. The American Heart Association and the American Stroke Association advise managing obesity for both primary [87] and secondary stroke prevention [88] in light of such results. The pleiotropic effects that a number of cytokines released by adipose tissue may have on vascular wall, inflammation, and insulin resistance are thought to be a plausible underlying mechanism relating obesity and stroke [89]. Adiponectin and hepatocyte growth factor are two examples of these adipokines, and low levels of adiponectin and high levels of hepatocyte growth factor have both been linked to an increased risk of stroke-related morbidity [90]. Adiponectin levels and the frequency of ischemic stroke, however, were not shown to be significantly correlated in other investigations [91]. Furthermore, in the morbid obese, higher stroke mortality was linked to both low and high adiponectin concentrations probably due to the transgene-mediated overexpression of adiponectin that causes morbid obesity due to decreased energy expenditure [92]. Additionally, according to a recent meta-analysis [93], individuals who were obese or overweight had a relative risk for ischemic stroke of 1.64 (95% CI: 1.36–1.99) and 1.22 (95% CI: 1.05–1.41), respectively, thus showing incrementally increased risk with increased BMI. Multivariate analysis of data from four cohorts involving 76,227 Chinese individuals revealed an increase of 2 kg/m^2 in baseline BMI resulting in 6.1% increase in the relative risk of total stroke [94].

5. Assessment of obesity as a comorbidity burden

Waist circumference is another clinically feasible measurement that may be used independently or in addition to body mass index BMI to assess weight-related health risk. The World Health Organization has identified sex-specific waist circumference values that signify increased health risk (≥80 cm for women, ≥94 cm for men) and substantially increased health risk (≥88 cm for women, ≥102 cm for men) [95, 96]. Waist circumference correlates well with BMI requiring only a tape measure to provides an estimate of abdominal fat. Abdominal fat is more strongly associated with health risk than fat stored in other regions of the body. Globally, the WHO obesity classification based on body mass index is the easily and generally adopted classification. Base on BMI it classifies obesity as >30 kg/m^2 for obesity, 25–29.9 kg/m^2 for overweight, 18.5–24.9 kg/m^2 for normal, and < 18.5 kg/m^2 as underweight and further classified obesity into 3 more categories of 30–34.9 kg/m^2 for obese-1, 35–39.9 kg/m^2 for obese 2 (super obese), and >40 kg/m^2 for obese 3 (morbid obesity) [97].

The World Obesity Federation (WOF) reiterated that obesity is a progressive disease process that can be chronic and relapsing in nature. Like other chronic illnesses, it's a progressive disease process where the diagnosis is based on some specific parameters such as high body mass index (BMI) value, where the higher the BMI, the more likelihood the devastating clinical consequences [22]. For example, patients with a BMI >30 reports more red flag signs such as shortness of breath and other specific disease symptoms concerning cardiopulmonary systems compared to patients within the normal BMI range [17].

6. Problem statement with obesity

The association between obesity and other life-threatening chronic diseases demands critical scrutiny, as obesity propensity for other diseases is estimated to be about 42% for both overweight and obese [11]. In the West, obesity is one of the most prevailing health problems associated with an increased tendency for development of several medical illnesses and premature loss of life [98], although this trend is fast germinating in the developing world too. Obesity predicaments caused a vast economic setback for medical facilities, and it created a massive financial meltdown for many nations, especially developing countries with poor health insurance and inadequate financial support. Besides, obesity is also linked with a reduced quality of life resulting from a number of associated diseases such as joint degenerative problems that cause pain and restrictions in carrying out daily activities and/or atherosclerosis that leads to Myocardial infarction and heart failure [98]. Obesity affects several portions of our bio-metabolic system from the heart to the liver, kidneys, joints, and reproductive system. It is associated with prevalence of multiple non-communicable diseases, such as type 2 diabetes, cardiovascular disease, hypertension, and stroke, and overall mental health in general. People living with obesity are also three times more likely to be hospitalized for infectious diseases like COVID-19 [99, 100].

At the psychosocial and economic level, obese individuals are less likely to obtain insurance, employment, promotion or enjoy personal relationships due to their quality-of-life predicament and health hindrances or even public stigmatization. Prevention especially and treatment of obesity is therefore now widely and critically recognized as the main priority for most healthcare governing bodies especially the WHO chapter of the United Nations [20]. The myriad of clinical implications of obesity make caring for obese patients a priority for most physicians, especially as mortality rises exponentially with increasing body weight [101, 102].

Psychosocial wellbeing is a measure of health or mental status in the form of quality of life. Although, the latter is a multidimensional notion that evaluates quality of life (QoL) and is associated with rising obesity level globally. QoL is an independent appraisal of both satisfactory and obnoxious features of life because the presumption is that people with higher BMI or weight are more probable to come up with an occurrence of certain mental situations [103]. Physical health in the form of phenotypic changes is a crucial contributing factor to overall quality of life [104]. Clinicians are increasingly coming to terms with the intricate association of obesity with quality of life because obesity is regarded as an important indicator and measure of quality of life. Obesity and psycho-mental disease such as anxiety-depressive disorder have a twisted and communal relationship, this is because obesity enhances the likelihood of getting a psychiatric diagnosis, and that the psycho-mental disorder may in turn further contribute to more weight gain and obesity [105]. Most of the available data from different research on the relationship between obesity and psychological diseases focused on the major depressive disorder, where the association has been proven to be strong [105]. Although the results of different research vary, the consensus is that there is a correlation between psychopathology and obesity for the majority of common or serious mental illnesses.

Comprehending the societal insights, demands, mindsets, perceptions, and preferences of individuals who are obese is essential because studies revealed societal observation and inclination more often than not have a negative perception towards people living with obesity [106, 107]. Often deem pessimistic due to low self-esteem and discrimination, body discrediting, and stigmatization. This could culminate in several adverse outcomes ranging from depression, anxiety, social phobia, declining medical support, and largely poor quality of life [106, 108]. These implanted unconstructive notions and trials encountered significantly derail or suppress their enthusiasm to manage their life situations thus, leading to a lack of devotion to weight-managing programs: lifestyle modifications, and pharmacological therapies. A detailed comprehension of the perceptions, attitudes, and preferences of the obese individuals is imperative to achieving an encouraging and societal-friendly atmosphere for the well-being of the people living with obesity.

People living with obesity are usually not satisfied with the outcomes from their healthcare provider visits especially if they feel that they were not given sufficient support from friends, or family members needed by them to achieve successful weight-reduction goals [109]. In fact, a study by Agüera et al. [110] showed that most people living with obesity feel that their physicians only accorded them limited time and do not view their health concerns from their own perspectives. These physicians are also reluctant to prescribe weight-lowering medications, they are over-aggressive in promoting strict lifestyle modification advice as the only ultimate way out. Painting pictures of them being at increased folds of developing life complications and poor quality of life.

7. Lifestyle-modifications, exercise and weight control inobesity

Early recognition and reduction of therapy barriers can conserve resources and increase the likelihood of long-term accomplishment, thereby safeguarding the patient from the medical illnesses and psychosocial, emotional and debilitative aftermath effects of excessive overweight/weight gain. Exercise is a crucial part of the behavioral therapy of obesity, along with dietary and lifestyle modifications. The components of these three therapeutic lifestyle changes or adjustment are essential initial stages in the prevention and treatment, but they are often omitted because of the complexity of their practical application [111]. Healthcare professionals that operate in an integrated team environment with a long-term horizon perspective are best able to deliver exercise along with calorie reduction, lifestyle modification, and in certain circumstances, weight loss medication and surgery, where clinical exercise physiologist play a significant role in this team [112]. The inclusion of clinical exercise physiologists in this type of programming is expected to continue to be successful considering that the prevalence of obesity in the United States and throughout the globe is not expected to decline noticeably in the near future [104]. This strategy makes it reasonable to manage, or perhaps eliminate the comorbidities associated with obesity while reducing the personal burden of obesity in a cost- and care-effective way..

As increase weight is associated with several factors from excessive food-intake to lack or inadequate daily mobile activity plus environmental and genetic factors, weight reduction and weight maintenance is undoubtedly a major task for individuals living with obesity. Both those with normal weights and those who are obese may benefit from increased physical exercise to improve their cardiovascular health status [113]. Regular bouts of aerobic exercise have been shown to lower blood pressure [114, 115], and visceral fat [114], the latter of which is linked to increased glucose tolerance and insulin sensitivity (in non-diabetic people) and glycaemic control (in type 2 diabetes patients). In another published study [116], investigators looked at 16 twin pairs with different levels of physical activity, they observed that sedentary twins had more visceral, hepatic, and intramuscular high-risk fat. The pairs with more physical activities had improved body composition and adequate metabolic parameters. Exercising 200 or more minutes per week was shown to more comparably weight loss than those who exercising less than 80 minutes per week in obese [117], such similar outcome was revealed in systematic reviews and meta-analyses published between 2010 and December 2019 [65].

In overall, a key to lessening overweight/obesity is early intervention, best even before conception. Balance and nutritious dietary intake in pregnancy, accompanied by exclusive breastfeeding for 6 months and beyond, perhaps until 2 years benefits all infant unobjectionably [118].

Therefore, public health approach to curtail overweight/obesity are crucial, but the evidence that even a modest weight loss is valuable if it is sustained makes management of obesity worthwhile and of paramount importance. A main mitigating factor to successful weight control therapy is time inadequacy, a commonly confronted barriers to obesity control [119]. Concerned individuals usually find it hard to create adequate time and space to take part in physical activity or to adopt healthy dietary routine or pattern. Because overweight/obesity being important global public health challenges, western and developing nations consider obesity as a chronic and progressive disease which demands resources and efforts as with other chronic illnesses and require lifelong management [120]. As such, there is no "quick fix" for overweight/obesity dilemma. Weight loss programs require great deal of lifelong commitment of dedicated lifestyle adjustment to achieve best weight reduction outcome, with tips on medical support and advice on how best to achieve and maintain a successful weight loss being offered by the medical experts and clinicians.

8. Conclusion

Consistently keeping an eye on one's BMI level, establishing a practical goal and engaging families and friends in the management routine and fight to lose weight are positive therapeutic steps, this is because, even losing what appears to be a modest quantity of weight, such as 3% or more of one's initial body weight and sustaining it for life-long, can significantly reduce the risk of obesity-related complications such as diabetes mellitus, osteoarthritis and cardiac diseases. If overweight/obesity is left unchecked, there is an increased risk of lifetime illnesses and disability by several folds. Additionally, overweight/obesity among the middle age is linked with poor index of quality of life and more detrimental effects in the older age group. Lastly, gender-wise, the overweight/obese women are more likely to develop depressive episodes and eating disorders, particularly the binge-eating disorder otherwise refer to as bulimia, especially if such individuals requires professional aid with their weight reduction plan. For these challenges and obstacles to weight reduction therapy or plan to be curtailed, appraisal and treatment are very crucial for successful reducing weight and eventual obesity-related chronic diseases.

9. Recommendation

Altogether, all nations must collaborate in global efforts to establish a better and healthy food ecosystem to avail everybody access to healthy diet. Pro-active measures restricting and regulating the sales of food and drinks high in fats food and drinks to children including introduction of appropriate taxing of sugary drinks. Government should provide cities and towns secured space or tarmac for safe exercising and recreation activities. Healthy diet and lifestyle practices should be taught as courses in schools to educate the pupils as well as public adverts to help families educate their children about a healthy habit. The global governing body that oversees the general wellbeing and world obesity crisis for humanity, the WHO, should intensify its supervision of the nationwide trends on overweigh/obesity prevalence, as well as creation of standard guidelines to tackling the prevention and treatment of overweight/obesity for all nations.

10. Limitation

The article does not touch on the heterogeneity of the several functions carried out by the neuronal network formed with other brain sections as there is a crucial links between the energy intake and expenditure effects mediated by distinctive neuronal subgroups as portrayed in distinctive brain waves monitoring.

Author details

Hafeez Abiola Afolabi[1], Zaidi Zakaria[1*], Salzihan Md. Salleh[2,3], Ewe Seng Ch'ng[4], Siti Norasikin Mohd Nafi[3], Ahmad Aizat Bin Abdul Aziz[5], Sameer Badri Al-Mhanna[6], Ahmad Adebayo Irekeola[7], Yusuf Wada[7] and Abubakar Bishir Daku[8]

1 Department of General Surgery, School of Medical Sciences, Hospital Universiti Sains Malaysia, Universiti Sains Malaysia USM, Kubang Kerian, Kelantan, Malaysia

2 Department of Pathology, School of Medical Sciences, Hospital Universiti Sains Malaysia, Universiti Sains Malaysia USM, Kubang Kerian, Kelantan, Malaysia

3 Department of Pathology, School of Medical Sciences, Universiti Sains Malaysia USM, Kubang Kerian, Kelantan, Malaysia

4 Advanced Medical and Dental Institute, Universiti Sains Malaysia USM, Kepala Batas, Penang, Malaysia

5 Department of Human Genome Centre, School of Medical Sciences, Health Campus, Universiti Sains Malaysia USM, Kubang Kerian, Kelantan, Malaysia

6 Department of Physiology and Exercise, School of Medical Sciences, Health Campus, Universiti Sains Malaysia USM, Kubang Kerian, Kelantan, Malaysia

7 Department of Medical Microbiology and Parasitology, School of Medical Sciences, Health Campus, Universiti Sains Malaysia USM, Kubang Kerian, Kelantan, Malaysia

8 Department of Human Physiology, School of Medical Sciences, Health Campus, Universiti Sains Malaysia USM, Kubang Kerian, Kelantan, Malaysia

*Address all correspondence to: doczakaria44@gmail.com

References

[1] Agofure O. Prevalence of obesity among adults in Issele-Uku, Delta State Nigeria. Alexandria Journal of Medicine. 2018;**54**(4):463-468

[2] World Health Organization. Health at a glance: Asia/Pacific. Measuring progress towards universal health coverage: Measuring progress towards universal health coverage. sixth edition of Health at a Glance Asia/Pacific, World Health Organization OECD summit 2020. Paris: OECD Publishing; 2020. DOI: 10.1787/26b007cd-en

[3] Simmonds M, Llewellyn A, Owen CG, Woolacott N. Predicting adult obesity from childhood obesity: A systematic review and meta-analysis. Obesity Reviews. 2016;**17**(2):95-107

[4] Anyabolu EN. Anaemia and its associated factors in patients attending a General Out-Patient Clinic in a tertiary hospital in Southeast Nigeria. International Journal of Medical and Biomedical Research. 2017;**6**(1):10-17

[5] Van Dyck D et al. International study of objectively measured physical activity and sedentary time with body mass index and obesity: IPEN adult study. International Journal of Obesity. 2015;**39**(2):199-207

[6] Robertson C. What the harm principle says about vaccination and healthcare rationing. Journal of Law and the Biosciences. 2022;**9**(1):lsac017

[7] Caldeira TCM, Soares MM, de Sousa TM, Veiga IPA, da Silva LES, Claro RM. The prevalence of risk and protective factors for noncommunicable diseases (NCDs) among Brazilian adults with pre-obesity and obesity. Obesities. 2022;**2**(3):317-325

[8] Maturo A, Setiffi F. Obesity, physical activity, and healthism. In: Wellness, Social Policy and Public Health. Bingley, England: Emerald Publishing Limited; 2022. pp. 21-32

[9] Afolabi HA et al. The relationship between obesity and other medical comorbidities. Obesity Medicine. 2020;**17**:100164

[10] D.-G. of W. Dr Tedros. World Obesity Day 2022 – Accelerating Action to Stop Obesity. Geneva: World Health Organization; 2022. pp. 1-2. Available from: https://www.who.int/news/item/04-03-2022-world-obesity-day-2022-accelerating-action-to-stop-obesity#

[11] Haththotuwa RN, Wijeyaratne CN, Senarath U. Worldwide epidemic of obesity. In: Obesity and Obstetrics. Colombo, Sri Lanka: Elsevier; 2020. pp. 3-8

[12] De Onis M et al. The W orld H ealth O rganization's global target for reducing childhood stunting by 2025: rationale and proposed actions. Maternal & Child Nutrition. 2013;**9**:6-26

[13] Yan SC et al. International defensive medicine in neurosurgery: Comparison of Canada, South Africa, and the United States. World Neurosurgery. 2016;**95**:53-61

[14] Marynak K, Gentzke A, Wang TW, Neff L, King BA. Exposure to electronic cigarette advertising among middle and high school students—United States, 2014-2016. Morbidity and Mortality Weekly Report. 2018;**67**(10):294

[15] McCartneySA,KachikisA,HuebnerEM, Walker CL, Chandrasekaran S, Adams Waldorf KM. Obesity as a contributor to

immunopathology in pregnant and non-pregnant adults with COVID-19. American Journal of Reproductive Immunology. 2020;**84**(5):e13320

[16] Lim HJ, Xue H, Wang Y. Global trends in obesity. Handbook Eating and Drinking Interdisciplinary Perspectives. 2020;**2020**:1217-1235

[17] Ogden CL, Carroll MD, Fryar CD, Flegal KM. Prevalence of Obesity among Adults and Youth: United States, 2011- 2014. Centers for Disease Control and Prevention CDC, United States of America USA. 2015

[18] Sultana R, Sissoho F, Kaushik VP, Raji MA. The case for early use of glucagon-like Peptide-1 receptor agonists in obstructive sleep Apnea patients with comorbid diabetes and metabolic syndrome. Life. 2022;**12**(8):1222

[19] Okati-Aliabad H, Ansari-Moghaddam A, Kargar S, Jabbari N. Prevalence of obesity and overweight among adults in the Middle East Countries from 2000 to 2020: A systematic review and meta-analysis. Journal of Obesity. 2022;**2022**:18. Article ID 8074837. DOI: 10.1155/2022/8074837

[20] World Health Organization. Regional Office for Europe. WHO European Regional Obesity Report 2022. World Health Organization. Regional Office for Europe. 2022. Available from: https://apps.who.int/iris/handle/10665/353747

[21] Seidell JC, Flegal KM. Assessing obesity: Classification and epidemiology. British Medical Bulletin. 1997;**53**(2):238-252

[22] Agha M, Agha R. The rising prevalence of obesity: Part A: Impact on public health. International Journal of Surgery and Oncology. 2017;**2**(7):e17

[23] Hou P et al. Association of Body Composition with pulmonary function in Ningxia: The China Northwest Cohort. Diabetes, Metabolic Syndrome Obesity Targets Therapy. 2022;**2022**:3243-3254

[24] Frellick M. US Adult Obesity Rate Jumped Over Last 20 Years. Medscape Logo, no. Medscape Medical News © 2018, [Online]. 2018. Available from: https://www.medscape.com/viewarticle/893957

[25] Chooi YC, Ding C, Magkos F. The epidemiology of obesity. Metabolism. 2019;**92**:6-10

[26] Cummins S, Macintyre S. Food environments and obesity—Neighbourhood or nation? International Journal of Epidemiology. 2006;**35**(1):100-104

[27] Lockyer S, Spiro A. Socio-Economic Inequalities in Childhood Obesity: Can Community Level Interventions Help to Reduce the Gap? London, United Kingdom: Wiley Online Library; 2019

[28] Van Zyl MK, Steyn NP, Marais ML. Characteristics and factors influencing fast food intake of young adult consumers in Johannesburg, South Africa. South African Journal of Clinical Nutrition. 2010;**23**(3):124-130

[29] van Hout G, van Heck G. Bariatric psychology, psychological aspects of weight loss surgery. Obesity Facts. 2009;**2**(1):10-15

[30] Hill JO, Pagliassotti MJ, Peters JC. Nongenetic determinants of obesity and body fat topography. In: The Genetics of Obesity. Florida, United States Of America USA: CRC Press; 2020. pp. 35-48

[31] Savage JS, Fisher JO, Birch LL. Parental influence on eating behavior:

Conception to adolescence. Journal of Law, Medical and Ethics. 2007;**35**(1):22-34

[32] Furlan A et al. Neurotensin neurons in the extended amygdala control dietary choice and energy homeostasis. Nature Neuroscience. 2022;**25**(11):1470-1480

[33] Kim MS et al. Prefrontal cortex and amygdala subregion morphology are associated with obesity and dietary self-control in children and adolescents. Frontiers in Human Neuroscience. 2020;**14**:563415

[34] Xia S et al. Cortical and thalamic interaction with amygdala-to-accumbens synapses. The Journal of Neuroscience. 2020;**40**(37):7119-7132

[35] Sahu B, Tikoo O, Pati B, Senapati U, Bal NC. Role of Distinct Fat Depots in Metabolic Regulation and Pathological Implications. Bhubaneswar, Odisha, India. 2022

[36] Islam T et al. Anti-inflammatory mechanisms of polyphenols in adipose tissue inflammation: Role of gut microbiota, intestinal barrier integrity and zinc homeostasis. The Journal of Nutritional Biochemistry. 2022;**2022**:109242

[37] Roji AYA, Paliwal M. Concept of Santarpana: A scientific analysis. Journal of Ayurveda Integrative Medical Science. 2021;**6**(3):84-93

[38] Cleary MP, Vasselli JR, Greenwood MR. Development of obesity in Zucker obese (fafa) rat in absence of hyperphagia. American Journal of Physiology Metabolism. 1980;**238**(3):E284-E292

[39] Reuter W, Ulbricht W. Adipocyte volume and count in obesity during weight reduction. Z. Gesamte Inn. Med. 1987;**42**(13):372-373

[40] Badawi A et al. Type 2 diabetes mellitus and inflammation: Prospects for biomarkers of risk and nutritional intervention. Diabetes, Metabolism Syndrome Obesity Targets Therapy. 2010;**2010**:173-186

[41] De Luca C, Olefsky JM. Inflammation and insulin resistance. FEBS Letters. 2008;**582**(1):97-105

[42] Stanley S, Wynne K, Bloom S. Gastrointestinal satiety signals III. Glucagon-like peptide 1, oxyntomodulin, peptide YY, and pancreatic polypeptide. American Journal of Physiological and Liver Physiology. 2004;**286**(5):G693-G697

[43] Huda MSB, Wilding JPH, Pinkney JH. Gut peptides and the regulation of appetite. Obesity Reviews. 2006;**7**(2):163-182

[44] Srivastava S, Rathor R, Singh S, Kumar B, Suryakumar G. Obesity: A risk factor for COVID-19. In: Coronavirus Therapeutics–Volume I. Delhi, India: Springer; 2021. pp. 195-210

[45] Chetambath R. Obesity, obstructive sleep apnoea, and metabolic syndrome: The fatal association. The Indian Practitioner. 2021;**74**(6):35-41

[46] Ofoegbu CKP, Manganyi RM. Off-pump coronary artery bypass grafting; is it still relevant? Current Cardiology Reviews. 2022;**18**(2):64-77

[47] Finkelstein EA. How big of a problem is obesity? Surgery for Obesity and Related Diseases. 2014;**10**(4):569-570

[48] Craig BM, Tseng DS. Cost-effectiveness of gastric bypass for severe obesity. The American Journal of Medicine. 2002;**113**(6):491-498

[49] Felisbino-Mendes MS et al. The burden of non-communicable diseases

attributable to high BMI in Brazil, 1990-2017: Findings from the global burden of disease study. Population Health Metrics. 2020;**18**(1):1-13

[50] Feigl AB, Goryakin Y, Devaux M, Lerouge A, Vuik S, Cecchini M. The short-term effect of BMI, alcohol use, and related chronic conditions on labour market outcomes: A time-lag panel analysis utilizing European SHARE dataset. PLoS One. 2019;**14**(3):e0211940

[51] Benjamin EJ et al. Heart disease and stroke statistics—2018 update: A report from the American Heart Association. Circulation. 2018;**137**(12):e67-e492

[52] Virani SS et al. Heart disease and stroke statistics—2020 update: A report from the American Heart Association. Circulation. 2020;**141**(9):e139-e596

[53] Hall JE, do Carmo JM, da Silva AA, Wang Z, Hall ME. Obesity, kidney dysfunction and hypertension: Mechanistic links. Nature Reviews. Nephrology. 2019;**15**(6):367-385

[54] Wang Y-X et al. Associations of birth weight and later life lifestyle factors with risk of cardiovascular disease in the USA: A prospective cohort study. EClinicalMedicine. 2022;**51**:101570

[55] Pi-Sunyer FX. The obesity epidemic: Pathophysiology and consequences of obesity. Obesity Research. 2002;**10**(S12):97S-104S

[56] Willett WC et al. Weight, weight change, and coronary heart disease in women: Risk within the 'normal' weight range. JAMA. 1995;**273**(6):461-465

[57] Mafort TT, Rufino R, Costa CH, Lopes AJ. Obesity: Systemic and pulmonary complications, biochemical abnormalities, and impairment of lung function. Multidisciplinary Respiratory Medicine. 2016;**11**(1):1-11

[58] Friedlander AH, Walker LA, Friedlander IK, Felsenfeld AL. Diagnosing and comanaging patients with obstructive sleep apnea syndrome. Journal of the American Dental Association (1939). 2000;**131**(8):1178-1184

[59] Murugan AT, Sharma G. Obesity and respiratory diseases. Chronic Respiratory Disease. 2008;**5**(4):233-242

[60] McNamara K et al. Targets and indicators for chronic disease prevention in Australia. Australian Health Policy Collaboration. 2019;**2019**

[61] Salome CM, King GG, Berend N. Pulmonary physiology and pathophysiology in obesity physiology of obesity and effects on lung function. Journal of Applied Physiology. 2010;**64**:206-211

[62] Al-Mhanna SB et al. Effectiveness of physical activity on immunity markers and quality of life in cancer patient: A systematic review. PeerJ. 2022;**10**:e13664

[63] Melrose J. The importance of the knee joint meniscal fibrocartilages as stabilizing weight bearing structures providing global protection to human knee-joint tissues. Cell. 2019;**8**(4):324

[64] Pal S. Mechanical properties of biological materials. In: Design of Artificial Human Joints & Organs. Boston, USA: Springer; 2014. pp. 23-40

[65] Bellicha A et al. Effect of exercise training on weight loss, body composition changes, and weight maintenance in adults with overweight or obesity: An overview of 12 systematic reviews and 149 studies. Obesity Reviews. 2021;**22**:e13256

[66] Mutalub YB et al. Gut microbiota modulation as a novel therapeutic strategy in Cardiometabolic diseases. Food. 2022;**11**(17):2575

[67] Adams DB. Biliary dyskinesia: Does it exist? If so, how do we diagnose it? Is laparoscopic cholecystectomy effective or a sham operation? Journal of Gastrointestinal Surgery. 2013;**17**(9):1550-1552

[68] Villaça Chaves G, Pereira SE, Saboya CJ, Ramalho A. Non-alcoholic fatty liver disease and its relationship with the nutritional status of vitamin A in individuals with class III obesity. Obesity Surgery. 2008;**18**(4):378-385

[69] Finer N. Medical consequences of obesity. Medicine (Baltimore). 2011;**39**(1):18-23

[70] Tahergorabi Z, Khazaei M, Moodi M, Chamani E. From obesity to cancer: A review on proposed mechanisms. Cell Biochemistry and Function. 2016;**34**(8):533-545

[71] Rose DP, Vona-Davis L. Biochemical and molecular mechanisms for the association between obesity, chronic inflammation, and breast cancer. BioFactors. 2014;**40**(1):1-12

[72] Dev R, Bruera E, Dalal S. Insulin resistance and body composition in cancer patients. Annals of Oncology. 2018;**29**:ii18-ii26

[73] Abreu MT, Peek RM Jr. Gastrointestinal malignancy and the microbiome. Gastroenterology. 2014;**146**(6):1534-1546

[74] Wolin KY, Carson K, Colditz GA. Obesity and cancer. The Oncologist. 2010;**15**(6):556-565

[75] Pischon T, et al. General and abdominal adiposity and risk of death in Europe. The New England Journal of Medicine. 2008;**359**(20):2105-2120

[76] Karra P et al. Metabolic dysfunction and obesity-related cancer: Beyond obesity and metabolic syndrome. Obesity. 2022;**30**(7):1323-1334

[77] Bhaskaran K, Douglas I, Forbes H, Santos-Silva I, Leon DA, Smeeth L. Body-mass index and risk of 22 specific cancers: A population-based cohort study of 5· 24 million UK adults. Lancet. 2014;**384**(9945):755-765

[78] Al-Mhanna SB et al. Effects of circuit training on patients with knee osteoarthritis: A systematic review and Meta-analysis. Healthcare. 2022;**10**(10):2041

[79] Calle EE, Thun MJ. Obesity and cancer. Oncogene. 2004;**23**(38): 6365-6378

[80] Kruger J, Bowles HR, Jones DA, Ainsworth BE, Kohl HW. Health-related quality of life, BMI and physical activity among US adults (⩾ 18 years): National Physical Activity and weight loss survey, 2002. International Journal of Obesity. 2007;**31**(2):321-327

[81] Dieli-Conwright CM et al. Effects of aerobic and resistance exercise on metabolic syndrome, sarcopenic obesity, and circulating biomarkers in overweight or obese survivors of breast cancer: A randomized controlled trial. Journal of Clinical Oncology. 2018;**36**(9):875

[82] Kroenke CH, Chen WY, Rosner B, Holmes MD. Weight, weight gain, and survival after breast cancer diagnosis. Journal of Clinical Oncology. 2005;**23**(7):1370-1378

[83] Holmes MD, Chen WY, Feskanich D, Kroenke CH, Colditz GA. Physical activity and survival after

breast cancer diagnosis. JAMA. 2005;**293**(20):2479-2486

[84] Chlebowski RT et al. Dietary fat reduction and breast cancer outcome: Interim efficacy results from the Women's intervention nutrition study. Journal of the National Cancer Institute. 2006;**98**(24):1767-1776

[85] Quiñones-Ossa GA, Lobo C, Garcia-Ballestas E, Florez WA, Moscote-Salazar LR, Agrawal A. Obesity and stroke: Does the paradox apply for stroke? Neurointervention. 2021;**16**(1):9-19

[86] Yatsuya H et al. Body mass index and risk of stroke and myocardial infarction in a relatively lean population: meta-analysis of 16 Japanese cohorts using individual data. Circulation. Cardiovascular Quality and Outcomes. 2010;**3**(5):498-505

[87] Goldstein LB et al. Guidelines for the primary prevention of stroke: A guideline for healthcare professionals from the American Heart Association/ American Stroke Association. Stroke. 2011;**42**(2):517-584

[88] Field T, Benavente O. Secondary prevention of stroke. Stroke Cerebrovascular Diseases. 2014;**2014**:163

[89] Rexrode KM. Emerging risk factors in women. Stroke. 2010;**41**(10):S9-S11

[90] Rajpathak SN et al. Hepatocyte growth factor and the risk of ischemic stroke developing among postmenopausal women: Results from the Women's Health Initiative. Stroke. 2010;**41**(5):857-862

[91] Ogorodnikova AD et al. High-molecular-weight adiponectin and incident ischemic stroke in postmenopausal women: A Women's Health Initiative Study. Stroke. 2010;**41**(7):1376-1381

[92] Nagasawa H, Yokota C, Toyoda K, Ito A, Minematsu K. High level of plasma adiponectin in acute stroke patients is associated with stroke mortality. Journal of the Neurological Sciences. 2011;**304**(1-2):102-106

[93] Strazzullo P, D'Elia L, Cairella G, Garbagnati F, Cappuccio FP, Scalfi L. Excess body weight and incidence of stroke: meta-analysis of prospective studies with 2 million participants. Stroke. 2010;**41**(5):e418-e426

[94] Wu Y et al. Determinants of developing stroke among low-income, rural residents: A 27-year population-based, prospective cohort study in northern China. Frontiers in Neurology. 2019;**10**:57

[95] Janssen I, Katzmarzyk PT, Ross R. Body mass index, waist circumference, and health risk: Evidence in support of current National Institutes of Health guidelines. Archives of Internal Medicine. 2002;**162**(18):2074-2079

[96] Lean MEJ, Han TS, Morrison CE. Waist circumference as a measure for indicating need for weight management. BMJ. 1995;**311**(6998):158-161

[97] Edelstein AI, Lovecchio F, Delagrammaticas DE, Fitz DW, Hardt KD, Manning DW. The impact of metabolic syndrome on 30-day complications following total joint arthroplasty. The Journal of Arthroplasty. 2017;**32**(2):362-366

[98] De Lorenzo A, Gratteri S, Gualtieri P, Cammarano A, Bertucci P, Di Renzo L. Why primary obesity is a disease? Journal of Translational Medicine. 2019;**17**(1):1-13

[99] Lighter J et al. Obesity in patients younger than 60 years is a risk factor for Covid-19 hospital admission. Clinical Infectious Diseases. 2020;**71**(15):896-897

[100] Popkin BM et al. Individuals with obesity and COVID-19: A global perspective on the epidemiology and biological relationships. Obesity Reviews. 2020;**21**(11):e13128

[101] Afolabi HA, Zakaria ZB, Hashim MNM, Vinayak CR, Shokri ABA. Body Mass Index and predisposition of patients to knee osteoarthritis. Obesity Medicine. 2019;**16**:100143

[102] Mitsakos AT, Irish W, DeMaria EJ, Pories WJ, Altieri MS. Body mass index and risk of mortality in patients undergoing bariatric surgery. Surgical Endoscopy. 2022;**2022**:1-9

[103] Todisco P, Donini LM. Eating disorders and obesity (ED&O) in the COVID-19 storm. Eating and Weight Disorders-Studies on Anorexia, Bulimia and Obesity. 2020;**26**(3):747-750

[104] Wadden TA, Webb VL, Moran CH, Bailer BA. Lifestyle modification for obesity: New developments in diet, physical activity, and behavior therapy. Circulation. 2012;**125**(9):1157-1170

[105] Kasen S, Cohen P, Chen H, Must A. Obesity and psychopathology in women: A three decade prospective study. International Journal of Obesity. 2008;**32**(3):558-566

[106] Schetz M et al. Obesity in the critically ill: A narrative review. Intensive Care Medicine. 2019;**45**(6):757-769

[107] Puhl RM, Himmelstein MS, Pearl RL. Weight stigma as a psychosocial contributor to obesity. The American Psychologist. 2020;**75**(2):274

[108] Abouzed M et al. Relation of depression and anxiety disorders in choosing obesity management in obese patients. International Journal of Preventive Medicine. 2022;**13**(10):13-136

[109] Pagoto S et al. Tweeting it off: Characteristics of adults who tweet about a weight loss attempt. Journal of American Medical Informatics Association. 2014;**21**(6):1032-1037

[110] Agüera Z, Lozano-Madrid M, Mallorquí-Bagué N, Jiménez-Murcia S, Menchón JM, Fernández-Aranda F. A review of binge eating disorder and obesity. Neuropsychiatrie. 2021;**35**(2):57-67

[111] Wadden TA, Butryn ML, Wilson C. Lifestyle modification for the management of obesity. Gastroenterology. 2007;**132**(6):2226-2238

[112] Wadden TA, Tronieri JS, Butryn ML. Lifestyle modification approaches for the treatment of obesity in adults. The American Psychologist. 2020;**75**(2):235

[113] Haskell WL et al. Physical activity and public health: Updated recommendation for adults from the American College of Sports Medicine and the American Heart Association. Circulation. 2007;**116**(9):1081

[114] Ross R et al. Exercise-induced reduction in obesity and insulin resistance in women: A randomized controlled trial. Obesity Research. 2004;**12**(5):789-798

[115] Whelton SP, Chin A, Xin X, He J. Effect of aerobic exercise on blood pressure: A meta-analysis of randomized, controlled trials. Annals of Internal Medicine. 2002;**136**(7):493-503

[116] Leskinen T et al. Leisure-time physical activity and high-risk fat: A longitudinal population-based twin study. International Journal of Obesity. 2009;**33**(11):1211-1218

[117] Jakicic JM, Winters C, Lang W, Wing RR. Effects of intermittent exercise

and use of home exercise equipment on adherence, weight loss, and fitness in overweight women: A randomized trial. JAMA. 1999;**282**(16):1554-1560

[118] Butte NF, Lopez-Alarcon MG, Garza C. Nutrient Adequacy of Exclusive Breastfeeding for the Term Infant during the First Six Months of Life. Texas, USA: World Health Organization; 2002

[119] Teixeira PJ et al. Exercise motivation, eating, and body image variables as predictors of weight control. Medical Science Sports Exercise. 2006;**38**(1):179-188

[120] WH Organization. Obesity: Preventing and Managing the Global Epidemic. Aberdeen, Scotland; 2000

Section 3

Recent Advances and Outcomes of Obesity Management

Chapter 6

Novel Anti-Obesity Pharmacotherapies

Firas Ghomraoui and Gitanjali Srivastava

Abstract

Obesity is a global disease that causes or exacerbates many severe weight-related complications such as diabetes, cardiovascular disease, and fatty liver. Though there are concerted efforts to combat this disease through several means, lifestyle therapy is still considered the mainstay treatment for obesity. Unfortunately, patients with obesity respond either modestly or unfavorable to lifestyle intervention alone. Although the classical definition of an AOM is a medication that can help reduce at least 5% of body weight over a period of 3 months, the more novel agents have far surpassed that. There are presently six major FDA-approved medications: orlistat, phentermine monotherapy, phentermine-topiramate, naltrexone-bupropion, liraglutide 3.0 mg, and semaglutide 2.4 mg. Great strides have been made in the development of more novel agents, particularly those that affect either the gut hormones controlling satiety or certain pancreatic hormones. In this chapter, we will discuss current and upcoming novel AOMs available to treat and manage obesity. We will explore the novel endocrine peptides that are presently market accessible and how treating to target is feasible in the new era of obesity medicine. Further clinical trials must be conducted to pave the way for safer and more effective agents with greater access and affordability.

Keywords: anti-obesity medications, medical weight loss, weight management, type 2 diabetes, amylin, pramlintide, semaglutide, liraglutide

1. Introduction

Obesity is a worldwide growing disease that causes or exacerbates weight-related medical conditions contributing to a growing economic burden on many of the healthcare systems around the world. Various diseases have been found to be caused primarily by obesity, including type 2 diabetes mellitus (T2DM), obstructive sleep apnea (OSA), cardiovascular disease (CVD), non-alcoholic fatty liver disease (NAFLD), and multiple cancers (namely liver, kidney, and gynecological cancers) [1]. As per the World Health Organization (WHO), obesity is categorized by Body Mass Index (BMI) of 30 and above, with overweight being between 25 and 30 [2]. Further classification as per the Center for Disease Control (CDC) guidelines include mild obesity (BMI between 30 and 35), moderate obesity (BMI between 35 and 40), and severe obesity (BMI more than 40) [3]. As per the WHO, as of 2016, there are 1.9 billion people who were classified as overweight around the world, with an extra 650 million with obesity [2]. This trend has been ballooning on an alarming rate with an incline in overweight and obesity rates, especially among children and adolescents from 4–18% globally between the years 1975 and 2016 [2].

Due to the rising prevalence and the major health consequences of obesity, there are unsurmountable efforts to combat this rising epidemic. Whereas adjunctive lifestyle therapy coupled with pharmacotherapy or surgical intervention remains a mainstay regimen for obesity treatment, several factors could impede clinically significant weight loss goals, rendering the journey tough for the majority of patients, including physical limitations due to injury (a possible consequence of obesity itself, nonetheless), socioeconomic status, and psychological factors. Therefore, focus on management has shifted towards a more wholesome approach that includes multidisciplinary intervention (dietary, exercise physiology, and clinical psychology referrals) to address barriers to care and other factors pertaining to decreased access to care. Furthermore, the advent of novel agents for treatment of obesity and subsequent Food and Drug Administration (FDA) approval to several of these agents recently have propelled these medications to the forefront of the fight against this debilitating disease.

As per the National Institutes of Health (NIH), the most updated guidelines to initiate medical treatment for obesity include a BMI that is greater than 30 or a BMI that is greater than 27 with a concurrent co-morbidity, such as T2DM or hypertension [4]. There are several definitions to what one considers significant weight loss. Weight loss at a total of 5% or more of baseline weight over a period of 3 months is considered clinically significant as per current studies, though more novel pharmacotherapies have now surpassed these goals [4]. Currently, there are six agents that are FDA approved for weight loss: orlistat, phentermine monotherapy, phentermine-topiramate, liraglutide 3.0 mg, naltrexone-bupropion, and (most recently) semaglutide 2.4 mg [5].

2. Older-generation AOMs

Orlistat, the first and oldest agent, is a pancreatic and gastric lipase inhibitor. One large prospective study done in 2004 showed a mean reduction in weight of 5.8 kg in patients taking orlistat compared to placebo (3 kg) over a period of 4 years [6]. However, its use has significantly decreased over the years to the well-documented side effects, which include kidney injury and kidney stones secondary to increase calcium oxalate formation in the renal tubules [7]. Phentermine-topiramate is the second FDA-approved medication and is consistent of a combination of phentermine, a central norepinephrine-releasing stimulant drug, and topiramate, an anti-migraine and anticonvulsant medication. One such randomized clinical trial, the SEQUEL study, showed an average of 9.3% and 10.5% reduction in weight in phentermine-topiramate half and full dose, respectively, compared to placebo (1.8%) over a period of 2 years [8]. Furthermore, the same study showed a reduction in diabetes development along with less side effects (which might include constipation, parathesias, and dry mouth) of this medication observed if administered over a longer period [8]. Naltrexone-bupropion (NB) is a combination medication consistent of naltrexone, and opioid antagonist medication, with bupropion, an anti-depressant medication [9]. A post-hoc analysis conducted by le Roux CW et al. in 2022 analyzing several clinical trials pertaining to this medication showed a consistent weight loss trajectory of 5–10% in all the patients taking NB compared to placebo [10].

Drug	Mechanism of action	Administration	Mean weight loss observed	Contraindications	ADRs
Orlistat	Pancreatic and gastric lipase inhibitor	120 mg orally three times/day	5.8 kg	Gallstones, malabsorption syndromes	Flatulence, diarrhea, bloating, kidney stones
Phentermine Monotherapy	Sympathomimetic amine	8 mg (short acting) 2–3 times/day, 15 mg once daily, 37.5 mg once daily	(10.0 +/– 1.2 kg)	History (hx) of cardiovascular disease, uncontrolled HTN, uncontrolled anxiety or bipolar disorder (manic type), MAOI use within the last 14 days	Insomnia, increased jitteriness, constipation, dry mouth
Phentermine/ topiramate	Combination of sympathomimetic amine and anti-epileptic medication	Start with 3.75/23 mg orally once daily for 14 days; increase to 7/46 mg once daily and monthly titration upwards to achieve weight loss	9.3%–10.5% mean weight reduction	Glaucoma, hyperthyroidism, or MAOI use within 14 days	Dyspepsia, insomnia, constipation, dry mouth
Naltrexone/ bupropion	Combination of opioid antagonist and antidepressant	Naltrexone 8 mg with bupropion 90mg; titrate upwards to two tablets twice daily	5–10% mean weight reduction	Seizure disorders, anorexia or bulimia nervosa, chronic opioid use, MAOI use within the past 14 days	GI symptoms, headaches, dry mouth
Liraglutide*	GLP-1 receptor agonist	Starts at 0.6 mg daily subcutaneous injection for 7 days, then up titrate by 0.6 mg daily every 7 days to reach maximum dose of 3 mg daily	Around 10% mean weight reduction	Family or personal hx of medullary thyroid cancer or multiple endocrine neoplasia (MEN)-2 syndrome	Nausea, diarrhea, hypoglycemia, decreased appetite, abdominal pain, suicidal ideation
Semaglutide*	GLP-1 receptor agonist	Start with 0.25 mg weekly subcutaneous injection, then up titrate every 4 weeks until maximum dose of 2.4 mg weekly	15.3% mean weight reduction	Family or personal hx of medullary thyroid cancer or multiple endocrine neoplasia (MEN)-2 syndrome	Nausea, diarrhea, hypoglycemia, decreased appetite, abdominal pain, suicidal ideation

Drug	Mechanism of action	Administration	Mean weight loss observed	Contraindications	ADRs
Tirzepatide*	Dual GLP-1 and GIP agonist	Start with 2.5 mg weekly subcutaneous injection, then up titrate by 2.5 mg weekly every 4 weeks until maximum dose of 15 mg weekly	20.9% mean weight reduction	Family or personal hx of medullary thyroid cancer or multiple endocrine neoplasia (MEN)-2 syndrome	Nausea, diarrhea, hypoglycemia, decreased appetite, abdominal pain, suicidal ideation
Cagrilintide*	Amylin analogue	Maximum dose of 4.5 mg weekly	10.8% mean weight reduction		Hypoglycemia
Cagrilintide-Semaglutide*	Combination of amylin analogue and a GLP-1 agonist	1.2 mg–2.4 mg weekly of cagrilintide with 2.4 mg weekly semaglutide	15.7–17.1% weight reduction	Family or personal hx of medullary thyroid cancer or multiple endocrine neoplasia (MEN)-2 syndrome	Nausea, diarrhea, hypoglycemia, decreased appetite, abdominal pain, suicidal ideation

Table 1.
Older generation and Novel anti-obesity pharmacotherapy summary.*

With greater understanding of the pathophysiology behind obesity, there have been gargantuan strides towards newer, more efficacious, and safer medications to induce weight loss compared to the medications in the older generation category. One such category of medications that are also FDA approved for weight loss include the Glucagon-like Peptide-1 (GLP-1) agonists. These medications, originally designed to be anti-diabetic medications, have shown consistent weight loss potential upon their use, even in non-diabetic patients [11]. As of this moment, the FDA has approved two medications of this category for weight loss: liraglutide and semaglutide. However, there are several barriers that could limit the use of these medications, most notably related to the cost of these medications and variable insurance coverage that patients could carry (**Table 1**).

3. Novel AOMs

3.1 Liraglutide and Semaglutide

Liraglutide is a daily injection and, at 3.0 mg daily, is used for weight loss (as opposed to 1.8 mg daily for T2DM management) [12]. A randomized clinical trial, conducted by Pi-Sunyer X et al. back in 2015, showed a total of 63.2% and 33.1% of all the participants losing at least 5% and 10% of their body weight, respectively as compared to placebo (27.1% and 10.6%, respectively) [12]. Furthermore, another study showed the odds of maintaining those rates of weight loss tripled with liraglutide vs. placebo [13]. Semaglutide is a similar medication from the same drug family but is administered as a weekly injection compared to liraglutide. This is currently the newest FDA-approved medication at 2.4 mg weekly injection. There are currently five clinical trials that looked at the efficacy of this medication for weight management in comparison to placebo that have been performed (named STEP 1–5) [14]. The latest clinical trial, named STEP 5, looked at the use of semaglutide 2.4 mg weekly for sustained long-term weight loss in patients who do not have T2DM over a 2-year period. In this trial, the patients who took semaglutide for weight loss reported a mean change in body weight of −15.3% compared to the placebo group (−2.6%; $P < 0.0001$) [15]. The most reported side effects with this medication were gastrointestinal symptoms, such as nausea and reflux (**Table 1**) [15].

3.2 Tirzepatide

Tirzepatide, a weekly-injectable medication that agonizes both the GLP-1 receptors and the glucose-dependent insulinotropic polypeptide (GIP). It was first developed as an anti-diabetic medication and has shown great efficacy of lowering HbA1c as was demonstrated in the SURPASS trials but was found to greatly induce weight loss too [16]. In fact, the latest SURPASS trial (named SURPASS-5) showed a mean body weight change from baseline of −5.4 kg, −7.5 mg, −8.8 mg, and 1.6 kg with tirzepatide 5 mg, 10 mg, 15 mg, and placebo, respectively, over a period of 40 weeks [16]. However, the most impactful clinical trial was just published recently by Jastreboff AM et al. In this trial, 2539 patients who were obese or overweight with one co-morbidity (excluding T2DM), were randomized into tirzepatide and placebo groups over 72 weeks. The results were quite spectacular, with a mean weight change of −20.9% on the highest dose of tirzepatide (15 mg weekly) compared to placebo (−3.1%; $P < 0.001$) [17]. Furthermore, 91% of those taking the highest dose of tirzepatide reported a more than 5% weight loss from baseline compared to placebo (35%; $P < 0.001$), fitting the criteria for clinically significant weight loss [17]. The most reported side effects mimic those of the GLP-1 agonists [17].

3.3 Cagrilintide

In addition to the gut hormones controlling satiety (such as GLP-1 and GIP), there are studies pertaining to mimicking pancreatic hormones such as amylin. Cagrilintide is a long-acting amylin analogue that is administered as a weekly injection [18]. In a randomized clinical trial performed by Lau DCW et al., patients who were either obese or overweight with one co-morbidity (excluding T2DM) were randomized into groups of cagrilintide, liraglutide, and placebo over a 26-week period. The patients who took cagrilintide (at maximum dose of 4.5 mg weekly) were shown consistently to experience higher weight loss (10.8%) in comparison to the liraglutide 3 mg daily group (9%) and placebo (3%); $p < 0{\cdot}001$ and p-0.03 respectively [18]. The most reported side effects with this medication include gastrointestinal symptoms such as nausea, constipation, and diarrhea [18].

Moreover, there has been growing interest in combinatory AOMs for greater efficacy and synergy and/or additive effects. Dual-action incretin cagrilintide + semaglutide 2.4 mg was most notably shown in a study conducted by Enebo LB et al. as recently as 2021 [19]. In this robust clinical trial, 96 patients were randomized to groups of cagrilintide at various doses vs. placebo (semaglutide 2.4 mg being given to all participants). The results were promising; the mean percentage bodyweight reduction was greater with cagrilintide 1.2 and 2.4 mg than with placebo over 20 weeks (15.7% weight reduction for cagrilintide 1.2 mg, 17·1% for cagrilintide 2.4 mg vs. 9.8% in the placebo groups). The side effects reported were mostly gastrointestinal symptoms by a third of the participants, with glycemic parameters improving in all groups [19]. Given the new findings in the literature pertaining to the latter medications, it is only a matter of time before tirzepatide, cagrilintide, and other combinations join the growing list of weight loss medications that are approved by the FDA for an obesity indication.

3.4 Setmelanotide

Another novel medication has achieved an orphan indication for rare genetic obesity. Setmelanotide, a melanocortin-4 receptor (MC4R) agonist, is one such example that acts upon energy homeostasis through the leptin-melanocortin pathway [20]. This medication is used to treat mono-genic obesity primarily, such as the ones that are due to congenital leptin receptor (LEPR) deficiency, a bi-allelic mutation causing a deficiency in pro-opiomelanocotin (POMC) deficiency or proprotein covertase subtilisin/kexin type 1 (PCSK1) deficiency [20]. Several phase 3 global clinical trials with setmelanotide reported consistent weight loss of more than 10% of the original body weight, with side effects being mostly hyperpigmentation followed by nausea and vomiting [20].

3.5 Updated bariatric surgery considerations

Presently, the most common bariatric surgery procedures performed are the vertical sleeve gastrectomy (VSG) and the Roux-en-Y gastric bypass surgery (RYGB). Both procedures are effective for weight reduction and treatment of type 2 DM, as several studies showed, with RYGB being superior to VSG in both aspects (although RYGB carried higher risk) [21, 22]. Recently, updated bariatric surgery guidelines were published by Eisenberg D et al. in 2022, thirty-one years after the previous guidelines [23]. The newer guidelines lower bariatric surgery criteria in patients to a BMI greater than 35 (irrespective of whether they have co-morbidities or not) or a BMI greater than 30 with a diagnosis of metabolic syndrome and significantly remove barriers to treatment [23]. These latest bariatric surgery guidelines stem from the clearer understanding of the underpinnings of energy metabolism and scientific progress leading to necessary revision of the original guidelines [23]. While bariatric surgery is able to achieve 30–35% weight loss, novel AOMs can be utilized as adjunctive pharmacotherapy pre- or post-operatively to target weight gain [24]. Thus, combinatory novel AOMs coupled with surgical intervention are likely to garner more evidence in the future.

3.6 Weight-related therapeutic targets

As we make scientific progress with >15% weight loss, improvement, or remission in metabolic dearrangements such as fatty liver, T2DM, and cardiovascular disease can now be feasible. Anti-diabetes medications, such as semaglutide, liraglutide, and the newer tirzepatide were serendipitously found to be novel AOMs. Consequential reduction in hemoglobin A1c levels occur with the use of these agents in patients with dual obesity-diabetes diagnosis. Several studies have been conducted comparing different agents with regards to their efficacy of lowering A1c targets; in one trial, tirzepatide was shown to be superior to semaglutide over a 40-week period (−2.24 percentage points vs. −1.86 percentage points respectively) [25]. Furthermore, another area of highlighted focus is cardiovascular disease where risk reduction is paramount [26–28]. There is now heavy focus on GLP-1s for such a role, as evidenced by the PIONEER, SELECT, and SUSTAIN trials. One trial evaluated the role of oral semaglutide with regards to cardiovascular outcomes, with overall reduction of cardiovascular events in the patients taking oral semaglutide vs. placebo (although statistically significant only for non-inferiority of oral semaglutide vs. placebo throughout the study) [28]. Additionally, non-alcoholic fatty liver disease (NAFLD) is a complication with growing incidence around the world, ostensibly tied to the rise of obesity. Again, GLP-1 s have shown great efficacy in this realm, as one meta-analysis of several clinical trials spanning several GLP-1 agents showcased an overall reduction of both absolute percentage of hepatic fat and serum liver enzymes over a median period of 26 weeks [29]. All in all, in addition to weight reduction, there are innumerable health benefits being observed because of the growing use of these novel anti-obesity medications.

3.7 Obesity medical devices

In addition to AOMs and surgical weight loss options, there are different anti-obesity medical devices. One such device is called Plenity, an oral, nonsystemic, super-absorbent hydrogel that has shown to reduce a mean weight loss of 6.4% compared to 4.4% in the placebo group over a 24-week period [30]. Another device that has been studied showcased a 3.68–4.52% drop in total body weight [31]. Further studies with regards to medical devices are underway to pave way for their wider introduction to combat this global epidemic.

4. Conclusion

In conclusion, there are great strides being made in the pharmacotherapeutic management of obesity, as a response to the growing dangers of obesity. Previously, clinically significant weight loss was thought to be greater than 5% or more; however, we are now entering a new era of obesity medicine where >15% might be the new target for weight loss intervention. With novel obesity pharmacotherapy in the horizon, greater awareness and more solid recognition of this malady as a disease requires unique attention from a socio-economic and policy-making level (involving the patient, the insurance companies, and the governing bodies) in order to ensure non-discriminatory access at reasonable prices.

Author details

Firas Ghomraoui[1,4] and Gitanjali Srivastava[1,2,3,4*]

1 Department of Medicine, Division of Diabetes, Endocrinology and Metabolism, Vanderbilt University School of Medicine, Nashville, TN, USA

2 Department of Surgery, Vanderbilt University School of Medicine, Nashville, TN, USA

3 Department of Pediatrics, Vanderbilt University School of Medicine, Nashville, TN, USA

4 Vanderbilt Weight Loss Center, Vanderbilt University Medical Center, Nashville, TN, USA

*Address all correspondence to: gitanjali.srivastava@vumc.org

References

[1] Rekha BK, Srivastava G, Reid TJ, Aronne LJ. Understanding the pathophysiologic pathways that underlie obesity and options for treatment. Expert Review of Endocrinology & Metabolism. 2004;**16**(6):321-338

[2] Obesity. https://www.who.int/health-topics/obesity#tab=tab_1. [Accessed October 27, 2022]

[3] Defining Adult Overweight and Obesity. https://www.cdc.gov/obesity/basics/adult-defining.html. [Accessed November 5, 2022]

[4] Prescription Medications to Treat Overweight & Obesity. https://www.niddk.nih.gov/health-information/weight-management/prescription-medications-treat-overweight-obesity. [Accessed November 5, 2022]

[5] Idrees Z, Cancarevic I, Huang L. FDA-approved pharmacotherapy for weight loss over the last decade. Cureus. 2022;**14**(9):e29262

[6] Torgerson JS, Hauptman J, Boldrin MN, Sjöström L. XENical in the prevention of diabetes in obese subjects (XENDOS) study: A randomized study of orlistat as an adjunct to lifestyle changes for the prevention of type 2 diabetes in obese patients. Diabetes Care. 2004;**27**(1):155-161

[7] Filippatos TD, Derdemezis CS, Gazi IF, Nakou ES, Mikhailidis DP, Elisaf MS. Orlistat-associated adverse effects and drug interactions: A critical review. Drug Safety. 2008;**31**(1):53-65

[8] Garvey WT, Ryan DH, Look M, Gadde KM, Allison DB, Peterson CA, et al. Two-year sustained weight loss and metabolic benefits with controlled-release phentermine/topiramate in obese and overweight adults (SEQUEL): A randomized, placebo-controlled, phase 3 extension study. The American Journal of Clinical Nutrition. 2012;**95**(2):297-308

[9] Sherman MM, Ungureanu S, Rey JA. Naltrexone/bupropion ER (Contrave): Newly approved treatment option for chronic weight Management in Obese Adults. P T. 2016;**41**(3):164-172

[10] le Roux CW, Fils-Aimé N, Camacho F, Gould E, Barakat M. The relationship between early weight loss and weight loss maintenance with naltrexone-bupropion therapy. Eclinical Medicine. 2022;**49**:101436

[11] Ard J, Fitch A, Fruh S, Herman L. Weight loss and maintenance related to the mechanism of action of glucagon-like peptide 1 receptor agonists. Advances in Therapy. 2021;**38**(6):2821-2839

[12] Pi-Sunyer X, Astrup A, Fujioka K, Greenway F, Halpern A, Krempf M, et al. A randomized, controlled Trial of 3.0 mg of Liraglutide in weight management. The New England Journal of Medicine. 2015;**373**(1):11-22

[13] le Roux CW, Astrup A, Fujioka K, Greenway F, Lau DCW, Van Gaal L, Ortiz RV, Wilding JPH, Skjøth TV, Manning LS, Pi-Sunyer X; SCALE Obesity Prediabetes NN8022-1839 Study Group. 3 years of liraglutide versus placebo for type 2 diabetes risk reduction and weight management in individuals with prediabetes: A randomised, double-blind trial. Lancet 2017;**389**(10077):1399-1409

[14] Kushner RF, Calanna S, Davies M, Dicker D, Garvey WT, Goldman B, et al.

Semaglutide 2.4 mg for the treatment of obesity: Key elements of the STEP trials 1 to 5. Obesity (Silver Spring). 2020;**28**(6):1050-1061

[15] Garvey WT, Batterham RL, Bhatta M, Buscemi S, Christensen LN, Frias JP, et al. STEP 5 study group. Two-year effects of semaglutide in adults with overweight or obesity: The STEP 5 trial. Nature Medicine. 2022;**28**(10):2083-2091

[16] Dahl D, Onishi Y, Norwood P, Huh R, Bray R, Patel H, et al. Effect of subcutaneous Tirzepatide vs placebo added to titrated insulin glargine on Glycemic control in patients with type 2 diabetes: The SURPASS-5 randomized clinical Trial. Journal of the American Medical Association. 2022;**327**(6):534-545

[17] Jastreboff AM, Aronne LJ, Ahmad NN, Wharton S, Connery L, Alves B, et al. SURMOUNT-1 Investigators. Tirzepatide once weekly for the treatment of obesity. The New England Journal of Medicine. 2022;**387**(3):205-216

[18] Lau DCW, Erichsen L, Francisco AM, Satylganova A, le Roux CW, McGowan B, et al. Once-weekly cagrilintide for weight management in people with overweight and obesity: A multicentre, randomised, double-blind, placebo-controlled and active-controlled, dose-finding phase 2 trial. Lancet. 2021;**398**(10317):2160-2172

[19] Enebo LB, Berthelsen KK, Kankam M, Lund MT, Rubino DM, Satylganova A, et al. Safety, tolerability, pharmacokinetics, and pharmacodynamics of concomitant administration of multiple doses of cagrilintide with semaglutide 2·4 mg for weight management: A randomised, controlled, phase 1b trial. Lancet. 2021;**397**(10286):1736-1748

[20] Clément K, van den Akker E, Argente J, Bahm A, Chung WK, Connors H, et al. Efficacy and safety of setmelanotide, an MC4R agonist, in individuals with severe obesity due to LEPR or POMC deficiency: Single-arm, open-label, multicentre, phase 3 trials. The Lancet Diabetes and Endocrinology. 2020;**8**(12):960-970

[21] Lager CJ, Esfandiari NH, Subauste AR, Kraftson AT, Brown MB, Cassidy RB, et al. Roux-en-Y gastric bypass vs. sleeve gastrectomy: Balancing the risks of surgery with the benefits of weight loss. Obesity Surgery. 2017;**27**(1):154-161

[22] Lewis KH, Arterburn DE, Zhang F, Callaway K, Wallace J, Fernandez A, et al. Comparative effectiveness of vertical sleeve gastrectomy versus Roux-en-Y gastric bypass for diabetes treatment: A claims-based cohort study. Annals of Surgery. 2021;**273**(5):940-948

[23] Eisenberg D, Shikora SA, Aarts E, Aminian A, Angrisani L, Cohen RV, et al. 2022 American Society for Metabolic and Bariatric Surgery (ASMBS) and International Federation for the Surgery of obesity and metabolic disorders (IFSO): Indications for metabolic and bariatric surgery. Surgery for Obesity and Related Diseases. 2022;**S1550-7289**(22):00641-00644

[24] Lautenbach A, Wernecke M, Huber TB, Stoll F, Wagner J, Meyhöfer SM, et al. The potential of Semaglutide once-weekly in patients without type 2 diabetes with weight regain or insufficient weight loss after bariatric surgery-a retrospective analysis. Obesity Surgery. 2022;**32**(10):3280-3288

[25] Frías JP, Davies MJ, Rosenstock J, Pérez Manghi FC, Fernández Landó L, Bergman BK, et al. SURPASS-2 Investigators. Tirzepatide versus

Semaglutide once weekly in patients with type 2 diabetes. The New England Journal of Medicine. 2021;**385**(6):503-515

[26] Ryan DH, Lingvay I, Colhoun HM, Deanfield J, Emerson SS, Kahn SE, et al. Semaglutide effects on cardiovascular outcomes in people with overweight or obesity (SELECT) rationale and design. American Heart Journal. 2020;**229**:61-69

[27] Quast DR, Nauck MA. Cardiovascular safety and benefits of semaglutide in patients with Type 2 Diabetes: Findings from SUSTAIN 6 and PIONEER 6. Frontiers Endocrinology (Lausanne). 2021;(12):645566

[28] Husain M, Birkenfeld AL, Donsmark M, Dungan K, Eliaschewitz FG, Franco DR, et al. Bain SC; PIONEER 6 Investigators. Oral Semaglutide and cardiovascular outcomes in patients with type 2 diabetes. The New England Journal of Medicine. 2019;**381**(9):841-851

[29] Mantovani A, Petracca G, Beatrice G, Csermely A, Lonardo A, Targher G. Glucagon-like Peptide-1 receptor agonists for treatment of nonalcoholic fatty liver disease and nonalcoholic Steatohepatitis: An updated Meta-analysis of randomized controlled trials. Metabolites. 2021;**11**(2):73

[30] Giruzzi N. Plenity (Oral Superabsorbent Hydrogel). Clinical Diabetes. 2020;**38**(3):313-314

[31] Shirin H, Richter V, Matalon S, Abramowich D, Maliar A, Shachar E, et al. Safety, tolerability and efficacy of a novel self-use biodegradable device for management of obesity. Obesity Science and Practice. 2019;**5**(4):376-382

Chapter 7

The Role of Dietary Interventions in the Management of Obesity

Asad Ullah, Muhammad Jamil and Johar Jamil

Abstract

The epidemic of obesity is taking over many parts of the world. The etiology of obesity is multifactorial; however, disordered energy balance regulation is a central feature. Obesity is managed by lifestyle changes alone or in combination with pharmacotherapy or bariatric surgery. Diet is an essential part of the primary and secondary prevention of obesity. Various dietary patterns have successfully induced acute weight loss, but no diet stands apart from others. Most agree that an ideal weight loss diet should be nutritionally adequate, safe, effective, affordable, and culturally admissible. Creating a negative energy balance is the underpinning theme across weight loss diets. Despite early weight loss, most individuals struggle to maintain weight long-term. Weight gain occurs due to a complex interaction of physiological, environmental, and psychological factors. Long-term weight management is influenced by lifelong conformity to low energy diet, lifestyle changes and ongoing support from family, friends, and healthcare professionals. Strategies should be implemented at the population level to prevent obesity. Policymakers, schools, businesses, healthcare providers, community leaders and individuals must unite at local, national, and international levels to fight the epidemic of obesity.

Keywords: low fat diet, low carbohydrate diet, Mediterranean diet, weight loss, fasting

1. Introduction

Obesity is a complex chronic disease with abnormal or excessive body fat that impairs health, increases the risk of long-term medical complications, and reduces life span. Obesity is associated with diabetes mellitus, hypertension, cardiovascular disorders, neurological conditions, e.g., Alzheimer's dementia, fatty liver disease, and certain cancers.

The prevalence of obesity has almost tripled globally between 1975 and 2016 [1]. It has reached to epidemic level and is expected to grow in the foreseeable future.

Patients with body mass index (BMI) >25 kg/m^2 or high abdominal girth (men >102 cm and women >88 cm) should consider weight loss. Other factors, such as a family history of obesity, fat distribution, obesity-associated comorbidities, and cardiovascular risk factors, influence obesity management.

Setting a weight loss goal is the first step. It should be realistic, achievable, and reasonable. Weight loss could be divided into two phases, i.e., initial rapid weight loss (up to 6 months) and slow maintenance phase (lifelong). Diet plays a substantial

Health outcome	Improvement after 10 kg weight loss
Blood pressure (BP)	10 mm Hg drop in systolic BP
	20 mm Hg drop in diastolic BP
Diabetes mellitus	50% drop in fasting glucose level
Lipid profile	10% drop in total cholesterol
	15% drop in LDL cholesterol
	30% drop in triglycerides
Mortality	20% fall in overall mortality

Table 1.
Advantages of 10 kg weight loss.

role in the early phase of weight loss. Research shows that a modest 5–10% weight loss improves lipid profile, glycemic control, and blood pressure [2] (**Table 1**). It is clinically safe and achievable; hence most weight loss programs aim for 5–10% weight loss in the acute phase.

Weight maintenance is more challenging. Adherence to a low-fat diet and regular physical activity determine success.

Lifestyle modification (including diet, stress management, sleep, and physical exercise) is the first line of treatment for class I (BMI 30–34.9 kg/m^2) & class II (BMI 35–39.5 kg/m^2) obesity. Most agree that diet plays a fundamental role in the etiology of obesity. The modern diet is rich in refined carbohydrates, animal fats, salt, additives, preservatives, and ultra-processed foods. All these attributes drive weight gain and obesity. Therefore, modifying diet alone or combined with other interventions could prevent or treat obesity.

Public health and social marketing shape the dietary patterns of the public. The current focus is on selecting healthy food and eating less. Unfortunately, this has created a misconception that calorie restriction is the only or main factor responsible for weight loss. Indeed, weight loss needs calorie restriction, but the mechanics of weight loss are far more complex than just calorie restriction.

2. Nutritional strategies for weight loss

Clinical and commercial weight loss programs have successfully used various dietary patterns. A common theme among weight loss diets is setting up a negative energy balance. Most weight loss programs target 0.5 to 1 kilogram weight loss per week. A calorie deficit of 500 per day or 3500 per week is sufficient to achieve this target. The recommended calorie intake for a patient is calculated by first calculating the resting metabolic rate and multiplying it by an appropriate physical activity factor to get the calories for weight maintenance. Then subtract calories to induce weight loss. A fixed-calorie diet is a relatively easy alternate approach. It recommends a predetermined daily calorie intake based on the calorie level, which caused weight loss in clinical trials.

After deciding the daily calorie intake limits the next step is to choose the appropriate diet. Patients and families should be actively involved in selecting the weight loss diet to ensure success.

Generic name	Popular examples	Dietary composition
Diets with variable macronutrient composition		
Low fat, high carbohydrate diet	Ornish, Pritkin, T factor and Fit or Fat diets	Carb- 45-65%
		Fat- ≤10–19%
		Protein- 10-20%
Low carbohydrate, high fat, high protein diet	Atkins, Stillman, Scarsdale & Carb addict's diet	Carb ≤20% (<100–125 g/day)
		Fat- 55-65%
		Protein- 25-40%
High protein, low carbohydrate diet	Sugar busters, Zone, South beach diets	Carb- 40-50%
		Fat- 30-40%
		Protein- 25-40%
Balanced low-calorie dietary patterns		
	Mediterranean diet	Carb- 35-40%
		Fat- 40-50%
		Protein- 12-20%
	DASH diet	Carb- 55-60%
		Fat- 20-30%
		Protein- 15-30%
	Portfolio	
	Nordic	
	Vegetarian	
	Low glycemic index	
	Paleolithic	
Calorie restricted diets	Low energy diet	900–1200 kcal/day
	Very low-energy diet - Optifast, Medifast diets & Health management resources program	<800 kcal/day
Food based approaches		
Intermittent fasting	Alternate day fasting 5:2 Time-restricted feeding	
Non-dieting approaches	Heath at every size	

Table 2.
Common dietary approaches for weight loss.

Table 2 summarizes some of the commonly used weight loss diets.

2.1 Macronutrient-based approaches for weight loss

The human diet comprises macronutrients, micronutrients, dietary fiber, and water. The macronutrients, i.e., carbohydrates, fat, and protein, are energy sources. Fat is the most energy-dense macronutrient and contains 9 kcal/gram. Carbohydrates and protein provide ~4 kcal/gram.

Macronutrient	Recommended proportion of energy from macronutrients/day for the healthy population
Carbohydrate	45–65%
Fat	20–35%
Protein	10–35%

Table 3.
Macronutrient reference values for the healthy population.

Dietary reference intake (DRI) provides reference values of nutrients in healthy populations. **Table 3** demonstrates the daily requirements of macronutrients for healthy individuals [3].

Macronutrient-based calorie-restricted diets have variable macronutrient composition. Keeping energy constant, increasing one macronutrient will result in a compensatory reduction of another macronutrient. For instance, a low carbohydrate diet will have relatively high fat and protein content.

2.1.1 Low-fat diet

A low-fat diet provides 20–25% of energy from fat, and a very low-fat diet yields 10–20% of energy from fat. The proponents of a low-fat diet hypothesize that reducing the most calorie-dense macronutrient, i.e., fat, could result in weight loss. However, this relationship is not as straightforward as it sounds. Epidemiologic data show increased body weight despite a reduction in overall fat intake.

A meta-analysis comparing low-fat and regular-fat diets reported greater weight loss (3–5 kg) in individuals with a 10% or more reduction in dietary fat intake [4]. Another review showed a dose-dependent decrease in weight with a low-fat diet. Every 1% reduction in fat was associated with 0.28 kg weight loss [5]. However, another meta-analysis failed to show a difference in weight loss with reduced and normal-fat diets [6].

Indeed high-fat intake is associated with weight gain; however, the weight loss effect is unclear within the low-fat range (<30% of total energy). A systematic review reported higher weight loss in higher fat quartiles within the low-fat range [7]. Weight loss achieved with a low-fat diet is comparable to other weight loss diets.

A low-fat diet is associated with reduced triglyceride levels. However, triglycerides could increase if high glycemic index (GI) carbohydrates replace fat. Interestingly, low GI carbohydrates or mono/polyunsaturated fat do not increase triglycerides [8].

It is a challenge to maintain a very low-fat diet long term.

2.1.2 Low-carbohydrate diet

This diet yield <45% of daily calorie intake from a carbohydrate source. But there is a lack of consensus on the exact amount of carbohydrates, making it difficult to compare outcomes of studies.

The low-carbohydrate intake suppresses insulin secretion, which decreases fat storage (carbohydrate-insulin model). The higher protein content enhances satiating and higher metabolic burn (200–300 kcal) due to the thermogenic effect. Although unproven, some also argue that the calories from proteins are less prone to be stored as fat than the equivalent caloric intake from a carbohydrate source.

A meta-analysis of 38 studies shows greater weight loss with a low carbohydrate diet than a high carbohydrate diet (16.9 vs. 1.9 kg respectively). However, randomized cross-over and randomized controlled trials did not report a significant difference in weight loss between low and high carbohydrate diet [9].

Carbohydrate-restricted diet enhances satiety and is easy to follow. Studies show increased insulin sensitivity and improvement in glycemic control with a high-fat diet [10]. Evidence confirms the benefits of a low-carbohydrate diet in type II diabetes mellitus [11]. They are famous for rapid weight loss, especially the ketogenic version.

Adverse effects include fatigue, nausea, halitosis, muscle cramps, dizziness, and headache. Most low-carbohydrate diets limit fruit and vegetables, which increases the risk of micronutrient deficiency, e.g., vitamin A, B1, B6, E, folic acid, calcium, potassium, and dietary fiber. Moreover, adherence to a very low-carbohydrate diet is a challenge.

Studies have raised concerns about increased cardiovascular risks with a low-carbohydrate diet, especially if the saturated fat intake is high. A meta-analysis confirmed an increase in low-density lipoprotein with a low carbohydrate diet, although high-density lipoprotein and triglycerides improved [12]. The high protein content of this diet could increase urinary calcium excretion, leading to osteoporosis. Renal impairment could ensue due to high acid load [13]. Gout could occur due to high purine content.

2.1.3 Ketogenic diet

Also called the keto diet is a very low carbohydrate diet that allows 20–50 grams of carbohydrates per day and induces ketosis. The ketogenic diet suppresses insulin secretion, thus switching the energy source from glucose to fat. The body attempts to keep glucose levels at an appropriate level through gluconeogenesis. However, as the body's ability to synthesize glucose declines, fat is mobilized and utilized to produce ketones through ketogenesis, which meet the body's energy demands. Ketosis suppresses appetite, food cravings and hunger [14], thus encouraging rapid weight loss. Notably, nutritional ketosis does not cause metabolic acidosis [15] as opposed to diabetic ketoacidosis.

Keto diets are popular in the weight loss industry but do not have full support from the medical community due to their side effects. **Table 4** shows the two commonly used ketogenic diets and their macronutrient contents.

A meta-analysis of 14 randomized trials with 12 months or more follow-up reported greater weight loss with a very low carbohydrate ketogenic diet [WMD: 0.91 kg (95% CI: −1.65 to −0.17) $p = 0.47$] compared to a low-fat diet [16].

Besides weight loss, the ketogenic diet has a therapeutic role in diseases such as epilepsy, non-alcoholic steatohepatitis, Alzheimer's disease, polycystic ovary syndrome, acne and certain cancers [17]. The exact mechanisms of therapeutic actions of the ketogenic diet are not fully understood; however, **Table 5** [17] illustrates the suggested mechanisms.

Types of Ketogenic diet	Carbohydrate	Fat	Protein
Low carbohydrate or keto diet	5–10%	65–80%	15–25%
Very low-energy diet	30–50%	5–35%	35–45%

Table 4.
Composition of ketogenic diets.

Disease condition	Proposed mechanisms
Epilepsy	• Affecting Mammalian target of rapamycin pathway • Reduced excitability of neurons • Direct anticonvulsant effect of ketones
Non-alcoholic steatohepatitis	• Enhancing hepatic insulin sensitivity • Reduced gluconeogenesis • Decrease intrahepatic triglycerides
Alzheimer's disease	• Improved neuronal excitability • Mitochondrial function • Protection against β-amyloid
Polycystic ovary syndrome	• Lowering of blood insulin level • Reduced insulin-like growth factor 1 (IGF-1)
Acne	• Reduced IGF-1
Cancers	• Reduced blood glucose and insulin levels

Table 5.
Proposed therapeutic mechanisms of keto diets in various medical conditions.

The long-term safety of the keto diet is yet to be confirmed. Epidemiological data correlate a low carbohydrate diet with high mortality [18]. The high-fat content of the keto diet is a concern. It adversely affects the gut microbiome, brain function, cardiovascular health, and metabolic profile. Furthermore, compliance with the ketogenic diet is a challenge.

The Keto diet should be used cautiously with sodium-glucose transporter 2 (SGLT2) inhibitors in diabetic patients [19] due to the risk of metabolic acidosis.

Most of the macronutrient-based dietary approaches result in significant weight loss in the short term. No macronutrient distribution has shown a meaningful advantage over others regarding weight loss or cardiometabolic benefits. POUND LOST study [20] compared four diets with macronutrient permutations in obese adults (BMI 25–40 (kg/m^2) in a free-living setting. Body weight and body fat (total, visceral, hepatic, and subcutaneous fat) were measured at 6 and 24 months. Regardless of the macronutrient composition, most participants lost body fat (12.4%), lean mass (3.5%), visceral fat (16.1%), subcutaneous fat (13.6%) and abdominal fat (13.8%) at 6 months. The critical determinants for weight loss were low-calorie density and high fiber intake. The structured eating patterns might have also contributed to weight loss. At 24 months, most participants regained 40% of the lost weight with no difference between the diets.

Quality of the macronutrients is equally crucial for health benefits. Eco-Atkin study [21] randomly assigned 47 overweight adults with hyperlipidemia to either a low carbohydrate (26%) vegan diet with high protein (31%) and fat (43%) from gluten, soya, vegetable oils and nuts or high carbohydrate lacto-ovo vegetarian diet (58% carbohydrate, 25% fat & 16% protein). Weight loss at 4 weeks was similar in both groups; however, total cholesterol, high-density lipoprotein ratio (−8.1%), low-density lipoprotein (−8.7%) and apolipoproteins B: A1 ratio (−9.6%) were significantly lower in the low carbohydrate group. Blood pressure was also lower in the low-carbohydrate vegan group. Twenty-three patients completed 6 months of follow-up in a free-living setting. Study participants lost further weight in both groups (−6.9 vs. −5.8 kg respectively). Lipid markers declined in both groups but more in the low carbohydrate vegan group than in the comparator group. This study highlighted the weight loss and cardiovascular benefits of a vegan diet over a vegetarian diet. Similarly, the Prospective Urban Rural Epidemiology (PURE) study reported low non-cardiovascular and all-cause mortality in individuals with high fruit, vegetable, and legume intake [22].

In clinical studies, restrictive dietary approaches show weight loss in the short term; however, increased hunger and dissatisfaction reduce their effectiveness and long-term sustainability.

2.2 Balanced low-calorie diets patterns

This approach focuses on the whole diet rather than targeting a specific macronutrient. Besides acute weight loss, it has beneficial cardiometabolic effects independent of weight loss. They are more satisfying and have a better consumer acceptance profile. Therefore, long-term compliance is better. A few common balanced macronutrient dietary patterns are discussed below.

2.2.1 Mediterranean diet pattern

The Mediterranean diet is popular in the Mediterranean basin but is adopted worldwide due to its favorable effects on cardiovascular risks and weight loss. Some of the longest-living people in the world have consumed the Mediterranean diet. Its ingredients are not homogeneous and vary from region to region. However, it is primarily a plant-based diet, which promotes a high intake of local fruit, vegetables, unrefined grains, nuts, legumes, and olive oil. Fermented dairy products, fish, and red wine are allowed in moderation, while a low intake of meat and meat products is recommended. Mediterranean diet is rich in dietary fiber, micronutrients, antioxidants, monounsaturated and omega-3 polyunsaturated fats. It is low in saturated fat. It offers more food diversity than restrictive diets.

Studies show contradictory results about the weight loss outcomes of Mediterranean diet. A systematic review of 21 epidemiologic studies provided mixed results regarding the effects of the Mediterranean diet on weight loss [23]. The mixed results could be due to heterogeneity, varied comparators, and inconsistent follow-up periods. A recent systematic review [24] of 5 randomized trials reported moderate weight loss (−3.8 to −10.1 Kg) beyond 12 months using the Mediterranean diet. The weight loss was superior to the low-fat diet but equal to the low-carbohydrate and American Diabetes Association diet. Further studies are needed to clarify the role of the Mediterranean diet in weight loss.

Regardless of weight loss, the antioxidant and anti-inflammatory properties of the Mediterranean diet have beneficial effects on the cardiometabolic profile. Some experts believe that the anti-atherogenic effect is related to bioactive constituents in Olive oil (esp. extra virgin oil) [25] rather the mono-unsaturated fat. PREvención con DIeta MEDiterránea (PREDIMED) study is the largest randomized controlled trial designed to assess the cardiovascular benefits of the Mediterranean diet [26]. The study randomly assigned 7447 participants with cardiovascular disease risk factors but no diagnosis of cardiovascular disease into three groups. Group 1 was assigned to a Mediterranean diet enriched with extra virgin olive oil (MD + EVOO), group 2 had a Mediterranean diet with nuts (MD + nuts) and group 3 was prescribed a low-fat diet. No restrictions were placed on energy intake. The unadjusted hazard ratio for the cardiovascular event was 0.70 (95% CI: 0.53–0.91) in MD + EVOO and 0.7 (95% CI:0.53–0.94) in MD + nuts compared to the control group. The risk of developing diabetes mellitus was lower in the MD groups. In June 2018, the PREDIMED study was retracted and republished due to errors in the randomization. However, study results and overall conclusion remained unchanged after re-analysis.

2.2.2 Dietary approach to stop hypertension (DASH) diet

DASH dietary pattern was introduced in the 1990s to prevent and treat hypertension. It advocates the intake of fresh fruit, vegetables, low or fat-free dairy and nuts. DASH diet recommends lower sodium intake (<1.5 g/day) and discourages using saturated fat and sweetened beverages.

A meta-analysis of the DASH diet reported a reduction in systolic and diastolic blood pressure by −7.4 and −4.4 mm Hg, respectively, compared to the comparator [27].

Besides its blood pressure-lowering effect, several studies have highlighted the favorable effects of the DASH diet on lipid profile, blood glucose and insulin resistance. It correlates with lower colorectal cancer risk and improved celiac and diverticular disease [28]. A meta-analysis of 13 studies revealed the weight loss effects of the DASH diet [29]. The weighted mean difference was −1.42 kg (95% CI: −2.03 to −0.82) in 8–24 weeks. The weight loss effect was more pronounced with a low-calorie DASH diet in obese individuals.

2.2.3 Portfolio pattern

It is a modified plant-based diet with cholesterol-lowering foods such as olive oil, nuts, legumes, pulses, barley, oats, psyllium, etc. Its role in weight loss is not clear.

2.2.4 Nordic pattern

It was launched in 2004 and comprised the traditional diet consumed in Nordic countries. It encourages the use of fruit, vegetables, spices, seafood, and unsaturated oils (Canola oil), while processed foods and red meat are discouraged.

A randomized study reported a mean weight loss of −4.7 kg with an ad libitum Nordic diet compared to −1.5 kg with an average Danish diet [30].

2.2.5 Vegetarian pattern

It is a heterogeneous diet emphasizing the consumption of plant-based food (e.g., fruit, vegetables, seeds, legumes etc.). A vegetarian diet is classified depending on the restrictions applied, but avoiding meat is a constant feature. Vegans avoid any food of animal origin, lacto-vegetarians can take dairy products, and lacto-ovo-vegetarians can take dairy and eggs.

The vegetarian diet is rich in polyunsaturated fatty acids (PUFA), monounsaturated fatty acids (MUFA), minerals, fiber, antioxidants, and plant sterols. All these ingredients favorably influence lipid profile and cardiovascular risks. The low-calorie density of vegetarian food encourages weight loss.

Multiple studies have shown weight loss with vegetarian diet [31].

2.2.6 Low glycemic index dietary pattern

The glycemic index is the blood glucose response to a defined amount of carbohydrate (50 grams) in a test food relative to a reference food (usually white bread).

The GI was primarily developed for managing diabetes mellitus; however, it has earned popularity in weight management.

Low GI foods positively modify blood glucose levels, insulin levels, blood pressure and lipid profile. Studies show an association between low GI food with higher weight loss (−1 to 3 kg) compared to other energy-restricted diets in the short term [32].

2.2.7 Paleolithic pattern

It is also called the 'old stone age' or 'caveman diet'. This pattern is based on the diet practiced by our ancestors 2 million years ago. Its ingredients vary from region to region but generally allow vegetable, fruit, pasture-raised or grass-fed meat, fish, poultry, and nuts. At the same time, processed foods, grains, legumes, and dairy are restricted.

The Paleolithic diet is nutritious; however, compliance is challenging due to the elimination of commonly consumed beverages and foods. Limited available research showed improved insulin sensitivity, lipid profile, weight loss and an association with lower frequency of certain cancers [33, 34].

2.3 Low-calorie dietary pattern

A low-calorie diet (LCD) allows 900–1200 kcal/day. LCD is popular for achieving rapid weight loss in a short time; however, weight regain is a concern. A systematic review reported a mean weight loss of 7–13 kg at 14 weeks [35]. The weight loss declined to 6–7 kg at 12 months and 3.5 kg at 2 yr. Most individuals were close to the pre-intervention weight at 5 yr., highlighting the difficulty in maintaining weight long-term. Interestingly, men attain higher weight loss with LCD than women (11.8 vs. 10.3% respectively) [36].

Furthermore, sustaining LCD is challenging due to its restrictive nature and low energy content. These diets pose the risk of micronutrient deficiency. Therefore, it should be supplemented with either multivitamins or fortified food.

The very low-calorie diet (VLCD) provides <900 kcal/day. It is best preserved for those with acute threatening health risks from obesity and where rapid weight loss could improve the outcomes. VLCD is used briefly before bariatric surgery to reduce the risk of complications.

Weight loss with VLCD is more impressive than with LCD. Ninety per cent of the patients accomplish more than 10% weight loss with VLCD vs. 60% of the patients with LCD. Weight loss slows substantially after 12 weeks due to a low resting metabolic rate and declining voluntary energy expenditure. Like LCD, the weight loss is more in men than in women (2–2.5 kg vs. 1.5–2 kg/week). Adding behavioral therapy and exercise to VLCD increases weight loss [37]. Studies show that VLCD could help in maintaining weight [37].

The Diabetes remission clinical trial (DiRECT) trial reported a high likelihood of diabetes mellitus remission with VLCD at 1 & 2 yr. follow-ups [38].

Some experts fear that the rapid weight loss with VLCD will follow rapid weight gain. But studies do not support this hypothesis [39].

VLCD is administered in a liquid formula based on milk or egg protein. It is supplemented with vitamins, fatty acids, and electrolytes to compensate for micronutrient deficiency. The protein content of VLCD is high (0.8–1.5 g/kg) to counter the lean mass loss.

Common side effects	Less frequent side effects
Dry skin	Electrolyte imbalance Cardiac arrhythmia
Fatigue, weakness, and lethargy	Seizures
Cold intolerance	Cholelithiasis
Dizziness	Osteoporosis
Nutritional ketosis	Anemia
Gastrointestinal effects - nausea, vomiting, constipation	Hair loss
Menstrual abnormalities	Skin thinning
	Muscle cramps
	Edema
	Nutrient deficiency

Table 6.
Side effects and complications of VLCD.

Table 6 summarizes the side effects of VLCD. Patients on VLCD therapy require close metabolic monitoring and should be administered only under the supervision of physicians with experience in this area.

VLCD is contraindicated in patients with a history of cardiovascular diseases, cardiac conduction abnormalities, recent myocardial infarction, type I diabetes mellitus, renal disease, hepatic disorders, burns, and pregnant or lactating women. Behavioral contraindications include acute psychiatric illness, substance abuse, major depression, bulimia nervosa, and bipolar disorder. Caution should be exercised if used in the elderly and pediatric population.

2.4 Food-based approaches

These dietary approaches recommend using specific foods such as fruit, vegetables, pulses (lentils, chickpeas, peas & beans etc.), nuts, whole grains, and dairy products. Evidence shows that these foods have a role in weight loss, maintaining body weight, and reducing cardiovascular risks.

2.5 FAD diets

The FAD diet is marketed as a quick fix for rapid weight loss in a short period. It is administered as a very restrictive diet or eating a few foods in an unusual pattern, such as eating only tomatoes. Such programs often make unreasonable claims that are not based on scientific evidence. A FAD diet could be harmful and should be discouraged.

2.6 Intermittent energy restriction

Fasting has been used for health benefits since the 5th Century BC [40]. In modern medicine, fasting in obesity management goes back to 1960s. Unfortunately, it went out of fashion due to serious adverse events. However, it has re-emerged as a therapeutic option recently. Besides weight loss, calorie restriction enhances insulin sensitivity, improves blood pressure, and reduces cardiovascular risks in animals. Furthermore, fasting correlates with cancer prevention and increased life expectancy in pre-clinical studies. The exact mechanisms for these changes are not fully understood. One hypothesis is the upregulation of the Sirtuins (SIRTs) signaling pathway. Sirtuin 1 (SIRT1) is an intra-nuclear molecule which deacetylates transcription factors involved in longevity and stress management. Calorie restriction upregulates SIRT1, which, in turn, reduces inflammation and increases insulin sensitivity [41]. SIRT1 reduces fat storage and resets the hormones linked with age pacing via the proliferator-activated receptor gamma pathway [42].

Fasting could be total prolonged fasting (TPF) or intermittent fasting (IF). TPF involves going without food for days. It is counterproductive for weight loss due to a compensatory decline in metabolic rate and physical activity. Moreover, it is associated with severe lean mass and micronutrient deficiency.

Intermittent fasting (IF) offers a sustainable and healthy alternative. It consists of fast and feast windows. Few or no calories are ingested during the fast, followed by ad libitum eating. IF is not a diet as such instead; it is about the timing of eating. In other words, any diet could be intercalated with IF.

Three common forms of IF are a 5:2 diet, alternate day fasting and time-restricted feeding (TRF). The 5:2 diet entails two fasts and five ad libitum feeding days per week. Alternate day fasting involves a day of fasting followed by an ad libitum eating day. TRF is the most popular form of IF. It implies an 8–10 hr. daytime feeding window followed by a 14–16 hr. fast (including overnight fast). The supporters of TRF hypothesize that eating food late at night may disrupt circadian rhythm, hormonal balance, glucose tolerance, reduce resting energy expenditure, and alter body temperature rhythms. Therefore, changing the eating time may improve the metabolism.

Fasting can reduce body weight by multiple mechanisms, i.e., calorie restriction, ketogenesis, interfering with the gut microbiome and establishing a feeding routine. A study compared a 5:2 diet with continuous energy restriction (1200–1500 kcal/day). The weight loss was comparable in the two groups (−6.8 ± 6.4 kg vs. −5.0 ± 7.1 kg, respectively) [43]. Another review of 40 studies reported that the IF caused 7–11 pounds of weight loss over 10 weeks; however, it was not superior to continuous energy restriction [44]. Furthermore, the adaptative responses to weight loss with IF were not different from continuous energy restriction.

Fasting remains an option in managing obesity, but further research is required.

2.7 Non-dieting approach

The traditional weight loss dietary approaches are predominately restrictive and fail to support weight maintenance. Non-dieting lifestyle approach is a popular alternative to the conventional weight-focused approach. The proponents of this weight-neutral approach believe that health is the outcome of behaviors independent of body weight. It focuses on a meaningful and fulfilling lifestyle. In a non-dieting program, food intake is guided by internal body cues, e.g., hunger and satiety [45], rather than external signals, such as meal time or events. Patients are encouraged to accept and respect their body size/shape at any weight. Health at Every Size (H@ES) is a program based on this philosophy. Besides intuitive eating, cognitive behavioral therapy and reasonable levels of physical activity administered in a non-restrictive way are other essential elements of H@ES.

Although the non-dieting approach is weight neutral, some studies have reported weight loss with this pattern. A randomized study compared a non-dieting eating pattern (1800 kcal/day) to a restrictive diet (1200 kcal/day). Weight loss was less in the non-dieting group than in the comparator group initially. However, at 12 months, greater weight loss was observed in the non-dieting group (10 vs. 4.5 Kg) than in the comparator [46]. Other studies revealed contradictory results; therefore, further research is needed.

The non-dieting approach has limitations and is not suitable for everyone. It is contraindicated in obese individuals fond of high-fat or high-sugar foods, those with extreme hunger signals, who consider eating large portions normal, and who lack the comprehension of healthy nutrition.

The non-dieting approach improves eating-related psychological disorders such as binge eating, depression, anxiety, and poor self-image [47].

3. Practical dietary interventions for weight loss

Regardless of the weight loss dietary approach, the following interventions could assist in achieving sustainable weight loss. It is essential to incorporate these strategies into daily routines to achieve the desired results.

3.1 Replacing high for low energy density foods

Studies show that people eat a consistent amount of food regularly. Therefore, diminishing the calorie density will lower the energy intake while eating satisfying meals.

The food energy density could be reduced by adding water-rich foods such as vegetables and non-starchy fruit. Another approach is reducing fat by using low-fat versions, e.g., grilled meat instead of fried meat or low-fat milk instead of full-fat dairy, without restricting the portion size. Besides quantity, the quality of fat also matters. Most dietary guidelines recommend substituting trans and saturated fat with monounsaturated and polyunsaturated fat.

Utilizing low-calorie dense foods at different meal courses could also help achieve sustainable weight loss. Studies indicate that selecting a large portion of low-energy-density food in the first course (starters) promotes satiety and helps lower the total calorie intake, e.g., low-calorie-dense salads and broth-based soups. Most of the energy intake occurs during the main course. Substituting high-calorie dense foods with low-calorie dense foods in entrée could support weight loss.

Food portion is another variable which influences energy intake. The larger the portion size, the higher the energy intake.

In a nutshell, reducing calorie density and controlling portion size promote weight loss.

3.2 Increasing satiety and adequate nutrients intake

3.2.1 Protein and fiber for fullness and satiety

An effective weight loss diet should satisfy hunger and induce satiety. Protein is the most satiating macronutrient. Protein intake reduces food intake and decreases the likelihood of snacking. Furthermore, protein preserves lean mass while on a low-calorie diet. It, in turn, keeps up basal metabolic rate supporting weight loss.

Dietary fiber comes from plant-based foods, but humans cannot fully digest dietary fiber. The undigested fiber confers a sense of fullness. Studies show that dietary fiber has a role in weight loss. Besides weight loss, it also has a role in preventing cardiovascular diseases, diabetes mellitus, stroke, and cancer (esp., bowel cancers) [48].

Dietary fiber exists in two forms, i.e., insoluble and soluble viscous forms. Insoluble fiber adds bulk to stool but does not impact the cardiometabolic profile. Soluble viscous fiber (found in oats, psyllium, barley, fruit, and vegetables) improves the cardiometabolic profile and glycemic control. DRI recommends an intake of 25–38 g of mixed fiber per day.

3.2.2 Reducing or eliminating the use of ultra-proceed foods

Ultra-processed food goes through multiple industrial processes (milling, molding) and has added ingredients which compromise its nutritional value. They are high in salt, sugar, and fat but deficient in fiber and micronutrients. For example, ice cream, chocolate, soft drinks, fries, sweetened breakfast cereals etc.

Several studies correlate the consumption of ultra-processed food with weight gain, risk of type II diabetes mellitus, cardiovascular diseases, cancers, depression, and overall mortality [49]. High glycemic load, poor nutritional value, displacement of healthful foods and poor gut-neuronal satiety signaling are some reasons for poor health outcomes.

A cohort study with almost 9 years of follow-up reported a 26% greater risk of weight gain in the higher quartile (6.1 servings/day) of ultra-processed food consumers compared to the lower quartile (1.5 servings/day) [50]. Eliminating or reducing ultra-processed food will support healthy weight and reduce the risk of diseases associated with such foods.

3.2.3 Using low calories beverages and water

Sugar-sweetened beverages (SSBs) add empty calories. It encourages weight gain by stimulating insulin secretion and probably activating the dopaminergic reward system in the brain. SSBs increase the risk of insulin resistance and cardiovascular risks independent of weight gain. The incidence of type II diabetes mellitus is higher among SSB consumers. Fruit drinks, sodas, sweetened carbonated drinks, cordials, sports drinks, and flavored drinks are examples of SSBs. Fruit juices are considered healthy and have nutrients; however, they are calorie dense and could cause weight gain if consumed in higher quantities.

Studies report a direct dose-response correlation between SSBs and long-term weight gain [51].

Substituting water or low-calorie sweetened beverages (tea, coffee, sparkling water etc.) for SSBs may promote healthy weight by reducing total calorie intake.

3.2.4 Substituting non-nutritive sweeteners for nutritive sweeteners

Nutritive sweeteners (NS) contain calories and promote weight gain; non-nutritive sweeteners (NNS) were introduced to replace NS.

NNS has zero or few calories. Logically, NNS use will reduce energy intake and weight. However, studies show mixed results. Prospective cohort studies report weight gain and increased risk of type II DM with NNS, while randomized controlled trials show beneficial effects of NNS on weight and type II DM [52]. This divide in studies conclusions is likely due to study design and differences in the controls. Controls in prospective studies are free living, and additional variables are not controlled for, while randomized trials control for additional variables. Further research is needed to provide insights into the benefits or harms of NNS.

4. Healthy dietary patterns tools

Selecting the right portion size is a challenge for most people. There is a need for tools that could guide the public in choosing the appropriate portion size.

Meal replacement (MR) or pre-packaged food is one such tool. It contains fixed calories (typically 200–300 kcal/serving). MR is available in various forms, such as snack bars, frozen meals, or shakes. It could be employed as a partial (as part of a low-calorie diet) or total meal replacement (as part of a very low-calorie diet).

In the first three to 4 months, partial meal replacement achieves 10–12% weight loss [53]. Systematic reviews and meta-analyses have demonstrated the efficacy of MR in achieving greater weight loss with partial meal replacement compared to conventional weight loss diets. MR has favorable effects on type II diabetes mellitus. The DiRECT study confirmed a 20-fold higher remission of diabetes mellitus at 12 months with total liquid meal replacement [38].

Portion control tools such as plates, bowels, serving spoons, cups, scales etc., could help limit food quantity; however, studies show these measures are insufficient. Poor compliance is a significant problem. Educating patients about proportion size is more effective. My Plate campaign is an example of a portion control education tool. It was launched by the United States Department of Agriculture (USDA) to promote healthy eating. It is an online tool which guides individuals about what and how much to eat.

Smartphone applications (apps) can support weight loss. Quite a few apps are already available in the market. Apps make weight loss activities measurable (by collecting data such as food intake, physical activity, distance traveled, sleep quality, heart rate, stress levels etc.), giving the consumer more control. The efficacy of apps in weight loss is controversial. Further studies are needed to validate their use in weight management. Apps could be used as an adjunct to other weight loss measures.

5. Maintaining weight loss

Many people succeed in losing weight, but only a few manage to keep it off. Some individuals regain a substantial amount of weight within 2 years, and most will retrieve all the weight lost in 5 yr. [54].

Why is weight maintenance so difficult? The initial rapid weight loss is followed by protective homeostatic changes, which resist further weight loss. Orixigenic hormone (ghrelin) increases while anorexigenic hormones (cholecystokinin, leptin, amylin, peptide YY and glucagon-like peptide 1) decrease [55]. Furthermore, the resting metabolic rate declines with weight loss. The muscles become more efficient in conserving energy. The net result of these changes is increased appetite and reduced energy expenditure resulting in weight gain [56]. Motivation drops as weight loss hits a plateau. The problem is further complicated by the easy availability of calorie-dense food and disinhibited eating habits.

Weight maintenance cannot be achieved only with diet; It requires a more holistic approach, including diet, physical activity, behavioral changes, and psychological support. Adherence to a low-calorie density diet and lifestyle modification are the keys to long-term success.

Research shows that individuals with ongoing support from friends, family, and healthcare professionals do better than those without help. The technology could be utilized to support sustainable weight loss. Genomics could help in selecting the appropriate diet for the right patient.

The National Weight Control Registry (NWCR) findings are an invaluable resource for weight maintenance. NWCR was established in 1994 to determine the characteristics of successful weight loss maintainers [57]. The database prospectively tracks over 10,000 individuals who have lost 30 pounds or more [mean 66 pounds (30–300 pounds)] and maintained it for at least 1 yr. [mean 5.5 yr. (1–66 yr)] [58].

The database has certain limitations. Firstly, it is not a prevalence study, and the sample is not random. Therefore, the results could not be extrapolated to the general population. Secondly, the participants self-identify themselves as eligible for the registry. Most of the information is self-reported, which is liable to bias. Thirdly, 80% of the participants are predominantly white females. Their mean age ranges between 45 and 49 yr. Despite its limitations, many studies support the NWCR findings.

The critical lessons learnt from the NWCR database are as follows: NWCR participants lost weight utilizing various interventions in the acute phase; however, there is limited variability in the strategies used for weight maintenance. Most consumed low fat (<30%), high carbohydrate and low energy diet to keep the weight off.

More than 90% of the participants used physical activity and diet to maintain weight. Most individuals do regular exercise (average 1 hour per day). Studies have revealed that physical activity preserves lean body mass regardless of weight loss which helps maintain a higher metabolic rate. Regular physical activity could also be a biomarker for compliance with other positive lifestyle modifications.

Seventy-eight per cent of the participants reported eating breakfast regularly. How breakfast contributes to sustainable weight loss is not clear. Perhaps eating breakfast may be more satiating than eating late in the day. Eating breakfast is correlated with lower BMI [59].

Almost all participants of NWCR weigh themselves at least weekly, and some even more frequently. Identifying increasing weight can act as an early warning sign that feeds back to institute corrective and preventative measures.

The dietary pattern of weight maintainers is consistent over the weekdays, weekends, and vacations all over the year.

Almost two-thirds of the individuals in NWCR spent less time in front of the television screen than the average American adult (≤ 10 hours vs. 28 hours per week). Watching TV is a passive activity, and most people also eat while watching TV. It is unclear what part of the energy balance contributes to weight gain, but watching TV is an independent marker of weight status regardless of the reason.

There are some exceptions to the behaviors mentioned above. Four per cent of the NWCR participants do not take breakfast; some individuals (<10%) take a low carbohydrate diet, and 9% do little or no exercise to maintain weight.

6. Conclusions

Obesity is a chronic disease which is associated with increased morbidity and mortality. The prevalence of obesity has increased globally.

It is managed by lifestyle modification alone or in combination with medications or surgery. Diet is an integral part of the primary and secondary prevention of obesity. There is no consensus on the best dietary approach for weight loss. However, most agree that an ideal weight loss diet should be culturally acceptable, palatable, satiating, low-energy-dense, nutritious, affordable, and sustainable. Most dietary guidelines recommend a high intake of whole grains, legumes, fresh fruit, vegetables, and nuts. Moderate consumption of unprocessed meat, eggs, and milk is encouraged, while refined sugars, high sodium, trans fat, and processed foods are discouraged. Patient and family involvement is essential in selecting the right diet plan for better compliance.

Most patients can achieve 5–10% weight loss with diet, but few can maintain it over an extended period. Management goals for weight maintenance are different; here, the emphasis is on long-term compliance with low calorie-dense, low-fat diet, physical activity, behavioral change, and psychosocial support.

Besides managing obesity at an individual level, tackling it at a population level is necessary. The existing measures for controlling obesity are inadequate. The public and private sectors need to step in and play their role. Weight management programs should be built into job plans, especially for high-risk jobs. Schools should embed healthy eating and physical activity in the curriculum. Food laws should promote healthy eating and exercise. There is room for improvement in the marketing regulations of unhealthy foods and drinks.

Acknowledgements

I would like to express my special thanks to my parents, wife, and children, who supported me in completing this work.

Conflict of interest

"The authors declare no conflict of interest." This work is not funded.

Notes/thanks/other declarations

None.

Author details

Asad Ullah[1*], Muhammad Jamil[2] and Johar Jamil[3]

1 University of Liverpool, Liverpool, UK

2 Retired General Practitioner, Peshawar, Pakistan

3 University of Swabi, Swabi, Pakistan

*Address all correspondence to: drasadullah99@hotmail.com

References

[1] WHO. Obesity and overweight. [updated 2023; cited 2023 01-03-2023]; 2021. Available from: https://www.who.int/news-room/fact-sheets/detail/obesity-and-overweight

[2] Knowler WC, Barrett-Connor E, Fowler SE, Hamman RF, Lachin JM, Walker EA, et al. Reduction in the incidence of type 2 diabetes with lifestyle intervention or metformin. The New England Journal of Medicine. 2002;**346**(6):393-403

[3] Trumbo P, Schlicker S, Yates AA, Poos M. Dietary reference intakes for energy, carbohydrate, fiber, fat, fatty acids, cholesterol, protein and amino acids. Journal of the American Dietetic Association. 2002;**102**(11):1621-1630

[4] Astrup A. The role of dietary fat in obesity. Seminars in Vascular Medicine. 2005;**5**(1):40-47

[5] Astrup A. The American paradox: The role of energy-dense fat-reduced food in the increasing prevalence of obesity. Current Opinion in Clinical Nutrition and Metabolic Care. 1998;**1**(6):573-577

[6] Pirozzo S, Summerbell C, Cameron C, Glasziou P. Should we recommend low-fat diets for obesity? Obesity Reviews. 2003;**4**(2):83-90

[7] Tobias DK, Chen M, Manson JE, Ludwig DS, Willett W, Hu FB. Effect of low-fat diet interventions versus other diet interventions on long-term weight change in adults: A systematic review and meta-analysis. The Lancet Diabetes and Endocrinology. 2015;**3**(12):968-979

[8] Hung T, Sievenpiper JL, Marchie A, Kendall CW, Jenkins DJ. Fat versus carbohydrate in insulin resistance, obesity, diabetes and cardiovascular disease. Current Opinion in Clinical Nutrition and Metabolic Care. 2003;**6**(2):165-176

[9] Bravata DM, Sanders L, Huang J, Krumholz HM, Olkin I, Gardner CD, et al. Efficacy and safety of low-carbohydrate diets: A systematic review. Journal of the American Medical Association. 2003;**289**(14):1837-1850

[10] Tay J, Thompson CH, Luscombe-Marsh ND, Wycherley TP, Noakes M, Buckley JD, et al. Effects of an energy-restricted low-carbohydrate, high unsaturated fat/low saturated fat diet versus a high-carbohydrate, low-fat diet in type 2 diabetes: A 2-year randomized clinical trial. Diabetes, Obesity & Metabolism. 2018;**20**(4):858-871

[11] Goldenberg JZ, Day A, Brinkworth GD, Sato J, Yamada S, Jönsson T, et al. Efficacy and safety of low and very low carbohydrate diets for type 2 diabetes remission: Systematic review and meta-analysis of published and unpublished randomized trial data. BMJ. 2021;**372**:m4743

[12] Mansoor N, Vinknes KJ, Veierød MB, Retterstøl K. Effects of low-carbohydrate diets v. low-fat diets on body weight and cardiovascular risk factors: A meta-analysis of randomised controlled trials. The British Journal of Nutrition. 2016;**115**(3):466-479

[13] Martin WF, Armstrong LE, Rodriguez NR. Dietary protein intake and renal function. Nutrition & Metabolism (London). 2005;**2**:25

[14] Abbasi J. Interest in the ketogenic diet grows for weight loss and type 2 diabetes. Journal of the American Medical Association. 2018;**319**(3):215-217

[15] Noakes TD, Windt J. Evidence that supports the prescription of low-carbohydrate high-fat diets: A narrative review. British Journal of Sports Medicine. 2017;**51**(2):133-139

[16] Bueno NB, de Melo IS, de Oliveira SL, da Rocha AT. Very-low-carbohydrate ketogenic diet v. low-fat diet for long-term weight loss: A meta-analysis of randomised controlled trials. The British Journal of Nutrition. 2013;**110**(7):1178-1187

[17] Paoli A, Rubini A, Volek JS, Grimaldi KA. Beyond weight loss: A review of the therapeutic uses of very-low-carbohydrate (ketogenic) diets. European Journal of Clinical Nutrition. 2013;**67**(8):789-796

[18] Seidelmann SB, Claggett B, Cheng S, Henglin M, Shah A, Steffen LM, et al. Dietary carbohydrate intake and mortality: A prospective cohort study and meta-analysis. The Lancet Public Health. 2018;**3**(9):e419-ee28

[19] Rosenstock J, Ferrannini E. Euglycemic diabetic ketoacidosis: A predictable, detectable, and preventable safety concern with SGLT2 inhibitors. Diabetes Care. 2015;**38**(9):1638-1642

[20] Sacks FM, Bray GA, Carey VJ, Smith SR, Ryan DH, Anton SD, et al. Comparison of weight-loss diets with different compositions of fat, protein, and carbohydrates. The New England Journal of Medicine. 2009;**360**(9):859-873

[21] Jenkins DJ, Wong JM, Kendall CW, Esfahani A, Ng VW, Leong TC, et al. Effect of a 6-month vegan low-carbohydrate ('Eco-Atkins') diet on cardiovascular risk factors and body weight in hyperlipidaemic adults: a randomised controlled trial. BMJ Open. 2014;**4**(2):e003505

[22] Miller V, Mente A, Dehghan M, Rangarajan S, Zhang X, Swaminathan S, et al. Fruit, vegetable, and legume intake, and cardiovascular disease and deaths in 18 countries (PURE): A prospective cohort study. Lancet. 2017;**390**(10107):2037-2049

[23] Buckland G, Bach A, Serra-Majem L. Obesity and the Mediterranean diet: A systematic review of observational and intervention studies. Obesity Reviews. 2008;**9**(6):582-593

[24] Mancini JG, Filion KB, Atallah R, Eisenberg MJ. Systematic review of the mediterranean diet for long-term weight loss. The American Journal of Medicine. 2016;**129**(4):407-15.e4

[25] Guo X, Tresserra-Rimbau A, Estruch R, Martínez-González MA, Medina-Remón A, Castañer O, et al. Effects of polyphenol, measured by a biomarker of total polyphenols in urine, on cardiovascular risk factors after a long-term follow-up in the PREDIMED study. Oxidative Medicine and Cellular Longevity. 2016;**2016**:2572606

[26] Estruch R, Ros E, Salas-Salvadó J, Covas M-I, Corella D, Arós F, et al. Primary prevention of cardiovascular disease with a mediterranean diet supplemented with extra-virgin olive oil or nuts. New England Journal of Medicine. 2018;**378**(25):e34

[27] Filippou CD, Tsioufis CP, Thomopoulos CG, Mihas CC, Dimitriadis KS, Sotiropoulou LI, et al. Dietary approaches to stop hypertension (dash) diet and blood pressure reduction in adults with and without hypertension: A systematic review and meta-analysis of randomized controlled trials. Advances in Nutrition. 2020;**11**(5):1150-1160

[28] Tyson CC, Nwankwo C, Lin PH, Svetkey LP. The dietary approaches to stop hypertension (DASH) eating pattern in

special populations. Current Hypertension Reports. 2012;**14**(5):388-396

[29] Soltani S, Shirani F, Chitsazi MJ, Salehi-Abargouei A. The effect of dietary approaches to stop hypertension (DASH) diet on weight and body composition in adults: A systematic review and meta-analysis of randomized controlled clinical trials. Obesity Reviews. 2016;**17**(5):442-454

[30] Poulsen SK, Due A, Jordy AB, Kiens B, Stark KD, Stender S, et al. Health effect of the New Nordic Diet in adults with increased waist circumference: A 6-mo randomized controlled trial. The American Journal of Clinical Nutrition. 2014;**99**(1):35-45

[31] Ivanova S, Delattre C, Karcheva-Bahchevanska D, Benbasat N, Nalbantova V, Ivanov K. Plant-based diet as a strategy for weight control. Foods. 2021;**10**(12):3052. DOI: 10.3390/foods10123052

[32] Thomas DE, Elliott EJ, Baur L. Low glycaemic index or low glycaemic load diets for overweight and obesity. Cochrane Database of Systematic Reviews. 2007;**2007**(3):Cd005105

[33] Frączek B, Pięta A, Burda A, Mazur-Kurach P, Tyrała F. Paleolithic diet-effect on the health status and performance of athletes? Nutrients. 2021;**13**(3):1019. DOI: 10.3390/nu13031019. Published 2021 Mar 21

[34] Whalen KA, McCullough M, Flanders WD, Hartman TJ, Judd S, Bostick RM. Paleolithic and mediterranean diet pattern scores and risk of incident, sporadic colorectal adenomas. American Journal of Epidemiology. 2014;**180**(11):1088-1097

[35] Glenny AM, O'Meara S, Melville A, Sheldon TA, Wilson C. The treatment and prevention of obesity: A systematic review of the literature. International Journal of Obesity and Related Metabolic Disorders. 1997;**21**(9):715-737

[36] Christensen P, Meinert Larsen T, Westerterp-Plantenga M, Macdonald I, Martinez JA, Handjiev S, et al. Men and women respond differently to rapid weight loss: Metabolic outcomes of a multi-centre intervention study after a low-energy diet in 2500 overweight, individuals with pre-diabetes (PREVIEW). Diabetes, Obesity & Metabolism. 2018;**20**(12):2840-2851

[37] Parretti HM, Jebb SA, Johns DJ, Lewis AL, Christian-Brown AM, Aveyard P. Clinical effectiveness of very-low-energy diets in the management of weight loss: A systematic review and meta-analysis of randomized controlled trials. Obesity Reviews. 2016;**17**(3):225-234

[38] Lean ME, Leslie WS, Barnes AC, Brosnahan N, Thom G, McCombie L, et al. Primary care-led weight management for remission of type 2 diabetes (DiRECT): An open-label, cluster-randomised trial. Lancet. 2018;**391**(10120):541-551

[39] Purcell K, Sumithran P, Prendergast LA, Bouniu CJ, Delbridge E, Proietto J. The effect of rate of weight loss on long-term weight management: A randomised controlled trial. The Lancet Diabetes and Endocrinology. 2014;**2**(12):954-962

[40] Britannica, The Editors of Encyclopaedia. "ṣawm". Encyclopedia Britannica, 1 Mar 2023. Available from: https://www.britannica.com/topic/sawm [Accesse: 5 March 2023]

[41] Madeo F, Carmona-Gutierrez D, Hofer SJ, Kroemer G. Caloric restriction mimetics against age-associated disease: Targets, mechanisms, and

therapeutic potential. Cell Metabolism. 2019;**29**(3):592-610

[42] Martin B, Mattson MP, Maudsley S. Caloric restriction and intermittent fasting: Two potential diets for successful brain aging. Ageing Research Reviews. 2006;**5**(3):332-353

[43] Carter S, Clifton PM, Keogh JB. Effect of intermittent compared with continuous energy restricted diet on glycemic control in patients with Type 2 diabetes: A randomized noninferiority trial. JAMA Network Open. 2018;**1**(3):e180756

[44] Seimon RV, Roekenes JA, Zibellini J, Zhu B, Gibson AA, Hills AP, et al. Do intermittent diets provide physiological benefits over continuous diets for weight loss? A systematic review of clinical trials. Molecular and Cellular Endocrinology. 2015;**418**(Pt 2):153-172

[45] Cummings S, Parham ES, Strain GW. Position of the American dietetic association: Weight management. Journal of the American Dietetic Association. 2002;**102**(8):1145-1155

[46] Sbrocco T, Nedegaard RC, Stone JM, Lewis EL. Behavioral choice treatment promotes continuing weight loss: Preliminary results of a cognitive-behavioral decision-based treatment for obesity. Journal of Consulting and Clinical Psychology. 1999;**67**(2):260-266

[47] Koller KA, Thompson KA, Miller AJ, Walsh EC, Bardone-Cone AM. Body appreciation and intuitive eating in eating disorder recovery. The International Journal of Eating Disorders. 2020;**53**(8):1261-1269

[48] Reynolds A, Mann J, Cummings J, Winter N, Mete E, Te Morenga L. Carbohydrate quality and human health: A series of systematic reviews and meta-analyses. Lancet. 2019;**393**(10170):434-445

[49] Elizabeth L, Machado P, Zinöcker M, Baker P, Lawrence M. Ultra-processed foods and health outcomes: A narrative review. Nutrients. 2020;**12**(7):1955. DOI: 10.3390/nu12071955

[50] Mendonça RD, Pimenta AM, Gea A, de la Fuente-Arrillaga C, Martinez-Gonzalez MA, Lopes AC, et al. Ultraprocessed food consumption and risk of overweight and obesity: The University of Navarra Follow-Up (SUN) cohort study. The American Journal of Clinical Nutrition. 2016;**104**(5):1433-1440

[51] Imamura F, O'Connor L, Ye Z, Mursu J, Hayashino Y, Bhupathiraju SN, et al. Consumption of sugar sweetened beverages, artificially sweetened beverages, and fruit juice and incidence of type 2 diabetes: Systematic review, meta-analysis, and estimation of population attributable fraction. BMJ. 2015;**351**:h3576

[52] Walbolt J, Koh Y. Non-nutritive sweeteners and their associations with obesity and type 2 diabetes. Journal of Obesity & Metabolic Syndrome. 2020;**29**(2):114-123

[53] Tsai AG, Wadden TA. The evolution of very-low-calorie diets: An update and meta-analysis. Obesity (Silver Spring). 2006;**14**(8):1283-1293

[54] Clinical Practice Guidelines For The Management Of Overweight And Obesity In Adults, Adolescents And Children In Australia 2013. Available from: https://www.nhmrc.gov.au/about-us/publications/clinical-practice-guidelines-management-overweight-and-obesity#block-views-block-file-attachments-content-block-1

[55] Lean ME, Malkova D. Altered gut and adipose tissue hormones in overweight and obese individuals: Cause or consequence? International Journal of Obesity. 2016;**40**(4):622-632

[56] Greenway FL. Physiological adaptations to weight loss and factors favouring weight regain. International Journal of Obesity. 2015;**39**(8):1188-1196

[57] Registry TNwc. Reserach findings. Available from: http://www.nwcr.ws/Research/default.htm

[58] Thomas JG, Bond DS, Phelan S, Hill JO, Wing RR. Weight-loss maintenance for 10 years in the National Weight Control Registry. American Journal of Preventive Medicine. 2014;**46**(1):17-23

[59] Sievert K, Hussain SM, Page MJ, Wang Y, Hughes HJ, Malek M, et al. Effect of breakfast on weight and energy intake: Systematic review and meta-analysis of randomised controlled trials. BMJ. 2019;**364**:l42

Chapter 8

Metabolic Outcomes in Obese Patients after Bariatric Embolization of the Left Gastric Vessel

Zaira Dzhamutdinovna Ramazanova,
Alexander Sergeevich Ametov and Evgeniya Yurievna Pashkova

Abstract

The prevalence of overweight and obesity is growing rapidly in the modern world. Currently more than 600 million people are obese, over 2 billion people are overweight. By 2025, according to World Health Organization experts (WHO), the number of people with obesity will increase almost twofold and will make from 30 to 50 percent of the population in economically developed countries. Embolization of the left gastric artery is an innovative, minimally invasive method of treating obesity, which allows to reduce body weight six months after its implementation by 17–18% on average. This technique, long used in emergency medicine as a method to stop gastric bleeding, has a new potential in the treatment of obesity. In this manuscript we present a pilot study examining the effects of bariatric embolization of the left gastric artery on the parameters of fat and carbohydrate metabolism in obese patients. We also present a case report illustrating the weight loss and the metabolic benefits of the left gastric artery embolization.

Keywords: embalization of the left gastic artery, obesity, grelin, leptin, high-molecular adiponectin

1. Introduction

Obesity has become the modern day epidemic affecting both developed and developing countries.

Data from numerous studies indicate that obesity has adverse metabolic effects on human health and is major cause for the development of diabetes mellitus, malignant neoplasms, cardiovascular diseases, as well as degenerative joint diseases, infertility, fatty liver disease, among others [1].

Obesity treatment comprises lifestyle interventions, including diet therapy, increased physical activity, psychotherapy as well as pharmacotherapy, and traditional bariatric surgery. It should be noted that the effectiveness of the conservative methods of treating obesity is quite limited compared to the results of bariatric surgery aimed at weight loss.

Bariatric surgery is by far the most effective strategy for achieving long-term weight loss. The use of bariatric surgery is justified in persons suffering from morbid obesity (body mass index above 40 kg/m^2), and in persons suffering from type 2 diabetes or other obesity-associated diseases - with an index over 35 kg/m^2. These surgical indications are particularly important given the lack of efficacy of conservative methods of treatment [2], Currently, the following types of bariatric surgery are most commonly used: gastric banding, sleeve gastroplasty, biliopancreatic bypass surgery and gastric bypass surgery [3].

Despite the fact that there is irrefutable evidence of the effectiveness of bariatric surgery over conservative methods of treating obesity, such operations like any surgical intervention, has many potential complications, and other health risks for patients and, moreover, surgical interventions do not always provide the desired results. These limitations of the current surgical interventions led to the emergence of new approaches in the fight against obesity, which would occupy their niche between standard bariatric surgery and conservative methods of treatment [4].

Bariatric embolization of the left gastric artery (ELGA), used for more than 40 years in emergency surgery to stop gastrointestinal bleeding, now is used as an innovative intervention of obesity management. During ELGA manipulation polyvinyl alcohol microspheres are introduced through the radial or femoral artery with a microcatheter, which subsequently creates ischemia of the gastric fundus that leads to the desired outcome: a decrease in the level of the hunger hormone ghrelin and a subsequent decrease in appetite [5].

The ghrelin hormone, the structure and function of which was first described by Kojima et al. in 1999, the 28th amino acid peptide that is produced by the endocrine cells lining the fundus of the stomach, remains today one of the known hormones that stimulates appetite. It is known that the level of ghrelin increases significantly during fasting and decreases after eating [6].

Ghrelin, having a powerful orexigenic effect and playing an important role in weight regulation, is a promising therapeutic target in bariatric surgery. Several studies [7–11] have demonstrated a significant decrease in weight as well as in ghrelin level after left gastric artery embolization [3, 12]. Thus, the definitive role of ghrelin in weight loss in obese patients after bariatric embolization is evident [3, 12, 13].

However, such studies have only examined the effect of bariatric embolization on body weight and ghrelin levels in obese patients. In this study we aim to evaluate not only weight reduction and ghrelin level after ELGA, but also to assess how changes in the level of the hunger hormone affect other hormones that regulate energy homeostasis and how to achieve weight stabilization after the initial weight loss with ELGA.

The aim of the current study is to evaluate the effect of bariatric embolization of the left gastric artery on the parameters of fat and carbohydrate metabolism in obese patients.

2. Materials and methods

A pilot study was conducted in the City Clinical Hospital n.a. S.P. Botkin in the Department of Endocrinology No. 59, which included 23 patients (10 men and 13 women, mean age 40.2 ± 10.6 years) with a diagnosis of morbid obesity (BMI > 40 kg/m^2) and obesity of the 2nd degree (BMI > 35 kg/m^2). In order to reduce body weight all the patients underwent surgical intervention in the form of bariatric embolization of the left gastric artery with polyvinyl alcohol microparticles 300–500 microns. Preoperative preparation included computed tomography of the aorta and its branches with contrast and administration of proton pump inhibitors.

During ELGA that is performed without anesthesia by transradial or transfemoral access, catheterization and angiography of the celiac trunk and left gastric artery were performed, followed by slow introduction of polyvinyl alcohol spherical particles with a diameter of 300–500 microns into the artery which led to the embolization of the left gastric artery. The duration of surgery is from 20 minutes to 1 hour.

The research work was approved at a meeting of the ethics committee of the Federal State Budgetary Educational Institution of Higher Education, Russian Medical Academy of Continuous Professional Education of the Ministry of Health of Russia dated on January 16, 2018 No 1.

Prior to the initiation of the study, each patient signed a written informed consent to participate in the study. All the patients before and after the bariatric embolization underwent an anthropometric examination including measurement of height, body weight, calculation of BMI, waist circumference (WC) as well as laboratory work including the determination of adiponectin, ghrelin and leptin. To assess carbohydrate metabolism, fasting plasma glucose, glycated hemoglobin, insulin, and HOMA-ir were also determined.

The severity of insulin resistance was determined using the HOMA-ir index, which was calculated using the formula HOMA-ir = (fasting glycemia (mmol/l) × IRI (immunoreactive insulin) (μU/ml))/22.5. The duration of the observation was 6 months, after which a follow up examination was carried out.

SPSS® statistical software version 21 was used to analyze our study data. The Wilcoxon test was used to assess the difference between the indicators before and after ELGA. Paired interrelations of indicators were determined by Pearson's rank correlation coefficient. The critical significance level (p) in the study was taken equal to 0.01. The results of the study are presented as M ± m, where M is the average value and m is the error of the mean.

3. Results

Preliminary results showed that 6 months after the bariatric embolization of the left gastric artery, a statistically significant decreases in all anthropometric parameters were observed: body weight decreased from 138 ± 33.2 kg to 114 ± 26 kg (18.5%, $p < 0.001$), BMI from 47.4 ± 9.3 kg/m^2 to 38.1 ± 7.4 kg/m^2 (19.6%, $p < 0.001$), WC index from 130.4 ± 9.7 cm to 115 ± 10.3 cm (9%, $p = 0.01$).

After ELGA, patients experienced a decrease in the hunger hormone and changes in the secretion of adipose tissue hormones. Previous studies have noted a decrease in weight and ghrelin level after ELGA [5, 6, 12]. Thus, the level of ghrelin decreased from 20.23 ± 4.6 to 2.09 ± 0.93 femtomol/μl (90% $p < 0.001$). The level of leptin, which is secreted in proportion to adipose tissue, decreased from 23.3 ± 4.9 ng/ml to 10.5 ± 3.7 ng/ml. (54% $p < 0.001$). At the same time, a correlation analysis was carried out between the change of body weight and the level of ghrelin, which has a positive correlation with the weight of patients after bariatric embolization ($r = 0.329$, $p < 0.01$).

In this study, the level of adiponectin was determined, which, according to the literature, is a key and universal marker of metabolic health [14]. It is known that the level of adiponectin is reduced in patients with visceral obesity and tends to increase with decreasing body weight [15]. The results of our study confirm these literature data: for example, 6 months after bariatric embolization, patients showed a

Parameter	Baseline	6 months	P-value
Body weight, kg	138.1 ± 33.2	113 ± 26	<0.001
BMI, kg/m^2	47.4 ± 9.3	38.1 ± 7.4	<0.001
WC, cm	130.4 ± 9.7	115 ± 10.3	<0.001
Fasting glycemia, mmol/l	6.9 ± 1.5	5.1 ± 0.7	<0.001
HbA1C, %	6.2 ± 1	5.3 ± 0.6	<0.001
Insulin, mcU/ml	15.6 ± 7.7	8.1 ± 0.7	<0.001
Adiponectin, mcg/ml	22.5 ± 8.1	20.1 ± 7.6	<0.001
Leptin, ng/ml	23.3 ± 4.9	21.2 ± 5.6	<0.001
HOMA-ir	4.5 ± 1.2	1.9 ± 0.32	<0.001
Ghrelin, femtomol/μl	20.23 ± 4.8	15.9 ± 5.2	<0.001

BMI, body mass index; WC, waist circumference etc.; HbA1C, glycated hemoglobin; Homa-ir, homeostasis model assessment of insulin resistance.

Table 1.
The dynamics of the studied parameters in patients with obesity before and after ELGA.

statistically significant increase in the average level of adiponectin from 22.5 ± 8.1 μg/ml to 42.4 ± 11 μg/ml (88.4%, $p < 0.001$).

As an example, we performed a correlation analysis between the change of adiponectin and body weight. Adiponectin negatively correlated with body weight of patients, the correlation coefficient after 6 months was ($r = -0.389$, $p < 0.01$). After ELGA, a positive change of carbohydrate metabolism was revealed.

The mean fasting glucose level initially before ELGA was 6.7 ± 0.9 mmol/l and by the sixth month it decreased to 5.3 ± 0.7 mmol/l ($p < 0.001$), the mean HbA1 level with an initial value of 6.2 ± 0.85% 6 months after the intervention showed a significant decrease to 5.5 ± 0.56% ($p < 0.001$), insulin initially −15.6 ± 7.7 μU/ml, after six months it decreased to 8.1 ± 0.7 μU/ml ($p < 0.001$), HOMA-IR index initially −4.5 ± 1.2, after 6 months of observation: −1.9 ± 0.32 ($p < 0.001$). The dynamics of the studied parameters of patients is presented in **Table 1**.

4. Discussion

Currently, the available therapeutic options as well as the surgical interventions to combat obesity are not fully effective. Several emerging therapeutic alternatives, are being evaluated in search of new, highly effective, yet safe methods of treating obesity.

Bariatric embolization of the left gastric artery appears to be an attractive therapeutic alternative that might become one of the most successful strategies in the fight against obesity while allowing control of energy consumption, affecting fat metabolism and significantly reducing the level of ghrelin, the hunger hormone.

The preliminary results of our pilot study, despite a small cohort of patients and the absence of a control group, showed that subjects who underwent bariatric embolization demonstrated a statistically significant weight loss 6 months after it was carried out by an average of 18–19%, a decrease in BMI, which was accompanied by a decrease in ghrelin by 90% and leptin by 54%, which are secreted in proportion to body fat mass.

It should be noted that previous studies evaluated only the changes of body weight measured in kg, BMI and ghrelin levels, but in our work we further evaluated other metabolic parameters and demonstrated how the level of ghrelin, which is the main underlying cause of weight loss in bariatric embolization, is associated with changes in other hormones that regulate energy homeostasis such as leptin, adiponectin [3, 12–14].

We also demonstrated at 6th month of observation, patients had a statistically significant increase in the average values of adiponectin by 84%, which has a negative correlation with body weight. An increase in the level of adiponectin was accompanied by a regression of metabolic changes in obese patients six months after the bariatric embolization, a decrease in body weight, an improvement in the sensitivity of peripheral tissues to insulin with the restoration of all parameters of carbohydrate metabolism and the prevention of many metabolic diseases, one of which is type 2 diabetes mellitus.

After the embolization of the left gastric artery in obese patients by 6 month, we demonstrated significant improvements in all indicators of carbohydrate metabolism: fasting glucose, HbA1c, insulin, HOMA-ir index.

While, future studies with long-term patients' follow-up will be required, our piolt data showed that bariatric embolization can become the very effective therapeutic intervention for obesity management in the short term, allowing not only to reduce body weight, but also to normalize carbohydrate metabolism and restore the hormonal function of adipose tissue.

Finally, we would like to present a clinical case of a patient who underwent embolization of the left gastric artery in order to reduce body weight.

Clinical case №1. Patient X., aged 48, was admitted to the Department of Endocrinology No 59 of the City Clinical Hospital n.a. S.P. Botkin with complaints of overweight, general weakness, fatigue, severe thirst, dry mouth and shortness of breath after walking a distance of less than 500 m.

Patient reported significant weight gain in 2011 after an accident resulting in left leg fracture which limited his physical activity. Subsequently, the patient noted an increase in weight of 10 kg per year. In 2016 he was diagnosed type 2 diabetes mellitus and oral hypoglycemic therapy with vildagliptin at a dosage of 50 mg was prescribed, followed by the addition of metformin at a dosage of 1000 mg twice a day. Also, the patient's condition was aggravated by arterial hypertension with an episodic increase to 220/120 mmHg, which he has been suffering from for 25 years.

On examination: height 178 cm, body weight 136 kg, BMI 42.9 kg/m^2.

On auscultation of the heart, the tones were muffled, rhythmic, no murmurs were heard, blood pressure was 140/85 mm Hg, the heart rate was 76 beats per minute. The frequency of respiratory movements was 16 per minute, with auscultation of the lungs, vesicular breathing was carried out in all parts of the lungs, there was no wheezing. The abdomen was enlarged due to subcutaneous fat, on the lateral surfaces of which striae were noted.

Biochemical profile revealed an increase in fasting glucose to 9.58 mmol/ml, glycated hemoglobin – 7.5%; insulin – 23.2 mU/l; C-peptide was 1642 pmol/l; HOMA-IR index (Homeostasis Model Assessment of Insulin Resistance) = 9.8; HOMA-β = 160.5. There were also high levels of uric acid up to 470 μmol/l, triglycerides up to 5.8 mmol/l, total cholesterol up to 6.7 mmol/l, LDL up to 3.5 mmol/l.

Ultrasound examination of the hepatobiliary system showed hepatomegaly, diffuse changes in the liver and pancreas of a lipomatous-fibrous nature.

The patient also underwent esophagogastroscopy, which revealed no contraindications to bariatric embolization of the left gastric artery.

Preoperative workup included ECG, echocardiography, radiography of the chest organs, ultrasound of the arteries and veins of the lower extremities, ultrasound examination of the kidneys and adrenal glands.

The patient was diagnosed with morbid obesity (BMI = 42.9 Kg/m^2). Diabetes mellitus type 2. The target level of glycated hemoglobin was less than 7%. Arterial hypertension of stage 3, a very high risk of cardiovascular complications. Dyslipidemia IIb. Hyperuricemia. Non-alcoholic fatty liver disease.

The indications for surgical treatment were determined for the patient, and subsequently, computed tomography of the aorta and its branches with contrast was performed to determine the anatomical variant of the gastric blood supply. Preparation for bariatric embolization also included the administration of the proton pump inhibitor drugs omeprozole 20 mg twice a day and sucralfate 1 g four times a day for a week before surgery.

In a planned manner in December 2017 in order to reduce body weight, the patient underwent surgical intervention in the form of X-ray endovascular bariatric embolization of the left gastric artery. The duration of the operation was 1 hour 10 minutes.

On the third day after the intervention, gastroscopy was performed, according to which no possible ischemic complications from the gastric mucosa were detected.

The examination of the patient before bariatric embolization, and after three days, 1 month, 3 and 6 months included the determination of body weight, BMI (Kg/m^2), fasting glucose, glycated hemoglobin, insulin, C-peptide, HOMA-IR, HOMA-β, as well as the level of ghrelin, leptin and high molecular weight adiponectin.

The results of the study showed that by the end of the first month after ELGA, the patient's weight decreased by 8% and amounted to 125 kg, by 3 months - by 11.7% (120 kg), by 6 months - by 17% (112 kg), and after a year body weight compared with baseline data decreased by 20.5% and amounted to 108 kg against 136 kg of initial weight. By the end of the 6th month of observation, BMI decreased to 35.3 kg/m^2 (−18.4% of the initial), and a year later decreased to 34 kg/m^2 (−20.7% of the initial).

It should be noted that we observed a decrease in the level of ghrelin and leptin by 6 months after ELGA and also should be especially emphasized, the significant increase in the level of high-molecular-weight adiponectin, which is a recognized universal marker of metabolic health (**Table 2**).

Date	Weight (kg)	BMI (kg/m^2)	Ghrelin (femtomol/μl)	Leptin (ng/ml)	Adiponectin (μg/ml)
At the time of admission	136	42.9	3.4	8.2	7.85
3 days after ELGA	134	42.2	2.55	7.7	11.59
1 month after ELGA	125	39.4	1.93	7.1	16.14
3 months after ELGA	120	37.8	1.5	4.7	16.92
3 months after ELGA	112	35.3	0.7	4.6	58.5
Δ % of the initial	−17.6%	−20.7%	- 73%	−43.9	+ 645%!!!

Table 2.
Changes in weight and hormonal profile in a patient with morbid obesity after ELGA.

Date	Fasting glucose (mmol/l)	HbA1c (%)	Insulin (μU/ml)	C-peptide (ng/ml)	HOMA-IR	HOMA-β
At the time of admission	9.58	7.5	23.2	4.9	9.8	76
3 days after ELGA	7.8	7.4	23.0	4.7	7.9	106
1 month after ELGA	5.17	6.9	15.6	4.1	3.5	186.8
3 months after ELGA	4.9	6.4	7.74	3.44	1.68	110.5
6 months after ELGA	4.8	6.1	7.5	3.2	1.6	115
Δ % of the initial	−49.4%	−18.6%	−67.6%	−34%	−75.3%	+51%

Table 3.
Changes of carbohydrate metabolism parameters in a patient with morbid obesity after bariatric embolization.

Date	Total cholesterol (mmol/l)	LDL (mmol/l)	HDL (mmol/l)	Triglycerides (mmol/l)	Uric acid (μmol/l)
At the time of admission	6.7	3.5	0.88	5.8	470
6 months after ELGA	3.17	1.86	1.4	2.13	367
Δ% of the initial	−52.5%	−46.8%	+93%	−63%	−21.9%

Table 4.
The dynamics of lipid profile parameters in an obese patient before and after ELGA.

The analysis of the parameters of carbohydrate metabolism after surgery showed a stable positive trend in the form of a stable decrease in fasting glycemia after 6 months to 4.8 mmol/l (−49.4% of the initial), the level of glycated hemoglobin to 6.1% (−18.6% of baseline), decrease in insulin to 7.5 μIU/ml (−67.6% of baseline) and C-peptide to 3.2 ng/ml34% of baseline), decrease in HOMA-IR to 1.6 (−75, 3% of the initial) and HOMA-β up to 115(+51%) (**Table 3**).

By the end of the sixth month of follow-up after surgery, we also obtained a significant decrease in the patient's uric acid level to 367 μmol/l (−21.9% of the baseline), a decrease in total cholesterol to 3.17 mmol/l (−52.5% of the baseline), as well as LDL up to 1.86 (−46.8%) and triglycerides up to 2.13 mmol/l (−63% of the baseline) (**Table 4**).

Author details

Zaira Dzhamutdinovna Ramazanova[1*], Alexander Sergeevich Ametov[1] and Evgeniya Yurievna Pashkova[1,2]

1 Department of Endocrinology, Federal State Budgetary Educational Institution of Further Professional Education "Russian Medical Academy of Continuous Professional Education" of the Ministry of Healthcare of the Russian Federation, Russia

2 Department of Endocrinology, Botkin Hospital, Moscow, Russia

*Address all correspondence to: zaira.ramazanova.92@list.ru

References

[1] Mohammed MS, Sendra S, Lloret J. Systems and WBANS for controlling obesity. Journal of Healthcare Engineering. 2018;**2018**:1564748

[2] Yashkov YuI, Karpova EV, Ametov AS. Bariatric surgery in the treatment of type 2 diabetes mellitus and obesity. Moscow: GEOTAR-Media; 2015. pp. 203-210

[3] Anton K, Rahman T, Bhanushali A. Bariatric left gastric artery embolization for the treatment of obesity: A review of gut hormone involvement in energy homeostasis. AJR Am J Roentgenol, 2016;**206**:202-210

[4] Rubino F. Metabolic surgery in the treatment algorithm for type 2 diabetes: A joint statement by international diabetes organizations. Diabetes Care. 2016;**39**:861-877

[5] Benso A, Gasanueva FF, Ghigo A. Ghrelin function in insulin release and glucose metabolism. Endocr Dev. 2013;**25**:135-143

[6] Kojima M, Kangava K. Ghrelin Discovery: A Decade After. Endocr Dev. Japan. 2013;**25**:1-4

[7] Arepally A, Barnett BP, Montgomery E, Patel TH. Catheter-directed gastric artery chemical embolization for modulation of systemic ghrelin levels in a porcine model: initial experience. Radiology. 2007;**244**(1):138-143

[8] Paxton BE, Alley CL, Crow JH, et al. Histopathologic and immunohistochemical sequelae of bariatric embolization in a porcine model. Journal Vasc Interv Radiol. 2014;**25**(3):455-461

[9] Bawudun D, Xing Y, Liu WY, et al. Ghrelin suppression and fat loss after let gastric artery embolization in canine model. Cardiovasc Intervent Radiol. 2012;**35**(6):1460-1466

[10] Gunn AJ et al. Is There a Role for Bariatric Embolization in the Tratment of the Diabetic Patient? J Vasc Interv Radiol. 2019;**30**(6):797-800

[11] Kipshidze N et al. A Novel Endoscopic Bariatric Procedure Results of an Experimental Stady. Obes Surg. 2016;**26**(12):3058-3065

[12] Weiss CR, Gunn AJ, Kim CY. Bariatric embolization of the gastric arteries for the treatment of obesity. Journal Vasc Interv Radiol. 2015;**26**(5):613-624

[13] Weiss CR. Short-term dynamics and metabolic impact of abdominal fat depots after bariatric surgery. Diabetes care. 2009;**32**(10)1910-1915

[14] Fiaschi T. Mechanisms of adiponectin action. International Journal of Molecular Sciences. 2019;**20**(2):2894

[15] Pankowska E, Szalecki M. Adiponectin as an adipose tissue hormone and its role in the metabolic syndrome and cardiovascular disease. Endokrynol Diabetol Chor Przemiany Materii Wieku Rozw. 2005;**11**(3):187-190